Mastering your Diabetes

(before diabetes masters you)

Janette Kirkham, RN, CDE, EMT

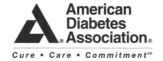

American Diabetes Association

Cure • Care • Commitment℠

Director, Book Publishing, John Fedor; *Associate Director, Consumer Books,* Sherrye Landrum; *Production Manager,* Peggy M. Rote; *Composition,* Circle Graphics, Inc.; *Cover Design,* Koncept, Inc.; *Printer,* Transcontinental Printing

Printed in Canada
1 3 5 7 9 10 8 6 4 2

The suggestions and information contained in this publication are generally consistent with the Clinical Practice Recommendations and other policies of the American Diabetes Association, but they do not represent the policy or position of the Association or any of its boards or committees. Reasonable steps have been taken to ensure the accuracy of the information presented. However, the American Diabetes Association cannot ensure the safety or efficacy of any product or service described in this publication. Individuals are advised to consult a physician or other appropriate health care professional before undertaking any diet or exercise program or taking any medication referred to in this publication. Professionals must use and apply their own professional judgment, experience, and training and should not rely solely on the information contained in this publication before prescribing any diet, exercise, or medication. The American Diabetes Association— its officers, directors, employees, volunteers, and members—assumes no responsibility or liability for personal or other injury, loss, or damage that may result from the suggestions or information in this publication.

♾ The paper in this publication meets the requirements of the ANSI Standard Z39.48-1992 (permanence of paper).

ADA titles may be purchased for business or promotional use or for special sales. To purchase this book in large quantities, or for custom editions of this book with your logo, contact Lee Romano Sequeira, Special Sales & Promotions, at the address below, or at LRomano@diabetes.org or 703-299-2046.

American Diabetes Association
1701 North Beauregard Street
Alexandria, Virginia 22311

Library of Congress Cataloging-in-Publication Data

Kirkham, Janette, 1966-
    Mastering your diabetes (before it masters you) / Janette Kirkham.
        p. cm.
    Includes bibliographical references and index.
    ISBN 1-58040-157-0 (pbk. : alk. paper)
    1. Diabetes—Popular works. I. Title.

RC660.4.K575 2003
616.4'62—dc21   2002043722

Contents

Preface

People tell me all the time that after living with diabetes for 27 years I must be used to it by now. I wish it were that simple. I may be used to blood monitoring, giving myself insulin injections, following a meal plan, and always thinking ahead about where I'll be and what I need to take with me. But time has not necessarily made having diabetes any easier. If anything, I am more tired of it. However, having diabetes for so many years has given me the chance to learn from experience and to discover creative ways to deal with this chronic illness. The opportunity to share these discoveries and "tricks of the trade" with patients has also helped me to manage my own diabetes better. It is my patients who have encouraged me to write *Mastering Your Diabetes (Before It Masters You)*.

Remember that all changes in your diabetes management need to be discussed with your physician. This book does not prescribe medical treatment. Instead, it explains creative ways to understand and live with this challenging disease. It is my hope that all who read this book will find the motivation and desire within them to rise to the challenge of diabetes—and master it.

Janette Kirkham, RN, CDE, EMT

Chapter 1

Congratulations— you have diabetes!

When you hear the words "You have diabetes," you experience many degrees of grief and emotion. You may experience **denial**, which helps sometimes to cushion the blow. You may tell yourself it was the Coke you drank on the way to your physician's office or the stress you have been under; or you think to yourself, "I'm only borderline, so I don't need to worry about it."

You may feel **anger** because you think that if you had known this was coming, you could have prevented it. Your self-talk may revolve around "I should have" statements. Maybe life has already dealt you enough trials to cope with, and one more like this just isn't fair. You may even feel angry at your parents or grandparents for the possibility that they passed diabetes on to you. Or you may feel angry at your physicians because they tell you that you have to change how you do things.

You may also find yourself trying to make bargains. **Bargaining** occurs when you make deals with yourself to try to make the diabetes go away. For example, you tell yourself you will never eat another thing with sugar in it, hoping this will make the diabetes go away.

Maybe you have noticed that you feel guilty, too. If you had eaten better and taken care of yourself, you think, this diabetes would never have happened. Or perhaps you had been told by your physician to lose weight, and you didn't do it.

Everyone diagnosed with diabetes feels **fear**—fear of finances, fear of needles, fear of complications, fear of failure, fear of the unknown, fear of being different, fear of having to do things differently, fear of high and low blood sugars, and fear of interference with day-to-day activities. What will happen to you?

Depression or **hopelessness** is common. You have been diagnosed with a chronic disease. Sometimes it feels as if you have been given a life sentence. If you don't have much emotional support from others, you may be wondering if you will be able to do all you need to do to take care of yourself. You will very likely feel sad at the loss of health. Furthermore, you probably feel overwhelmed and lost because you do not know the impact diabetes will have on your life. You do not know where or how to get started to take care of yourself, nor do you know whom to turn to for direction to overcome your loss of control.

A feeling of **acceptance** eventually comes when you finally realize the diabetes is yours. You recognize that it is not going away no matter how sad or angry you feel, or how much bargaining you do. Eventually you decide to find out what to do with it. This acceptance comes in bits and pieces. It is a stage that you will have to recommit to over and over. Even after all these years, I still have days when I do not want to think or talk about diabetes, and that can be a real challenge, since I work in a diabetes clinic. Thinking in terms of taking "one day at a time" when things are rough helps you achieve acceptance. Acceptance is also not all-encompassing. You may find that you accept certain parts of your diabetes, while you still avoid or deny other parts of the disease.

And believe it or not, some people sooner or later feel a **sense of relief**, for at least a couple of reasons. For one thing, you may have thought the diabetes was going to be much, much worse to deal with than it has turned out to be. Or the relief may come because you finally have an answer to why you don't feel well.

Every week, I hear patients say that they felt frustrated that they did not feel well but could not find an explanation for it. One of the most frustrating aspects of adult-onset (type 2) diabetes is trying to convince a physician you do not feel well when you look perfectly fine.

These emotions come and go differently for each person, and there is no correct order in which to proceed through them. You will find that with new challenges from your diabetes, or at the onset of a new complication, your grief process will start again, and you will likely cycle through them all over again.

If you have felt these or other emotions, you are normal. Recognizing the emotional impact of diabetes is every bit as important as taking care of the physical aspect of it. As a matter a fact, people often have to address the emotional issues before they can address their medical needs. For this reason, I try not to educate people on the same day they have been diagnosed. You need to cope with your own emotions first, then with the diabetes.

The goal is to not get stuck in a stage, because this can certainly thwart self-care. You have the right to feel your anger for as long as you want. Unfortunately, staying angry does not leave you much energy for anything else. It takes a balance of emotional, educational, and medical support to manage your diabetes effectively.

I have tried to cover each of these areas with tricks that have worked for me. I find that when I do not want to understand something, my mind makes it out to be more difficult or challenging than it really is. Diabetes is like that. I am not going to tell you that diabetes management is easy, because it is not. But with knowledge and insight about diabetes, you gain tools to help you conquer fears and answer questions. Many books on diabetes tell you what not to do and then give you a whole list of things to do. I want to give you some ideas on *how* to do these things. Again, diabetes management is not easy. But it can be made easier with tricks of the trade from someone who has "been there, done that." That is my hope for you as you read this book.

Chapter 2

What's supposed to be happening that isn't?

So what is diabetes? I have heard diabetes explained a dozen different ways. But most definitions are technical and hard to understand. It doesn't have to be that way. To understand diabetes, you first need to understand the body's metabolic process—what is supposed to be happening to the food that you eat. Once you know what should be occurring in your body but is not happening, it will be easier to understand diabetes and what you need to do to manage it. This knowledge helps you understand what your new job is, what your goals are, and how to achieve them.

Metabolism involves all the processes your body goes through to turn food into energy. Proper metabolism could not happen without insulin from the pancreas. When working correctly, the pancreas is responsible for many components of metabolism, most importantly blood sugar control. The pancreas does three things that directly affect blood sugar levels.

First of all, when you eat, the pancreas releases **digestive enzymes**. These enzymes break the food down into extremely small pieces of nutrition, namely fats, proteins, and sugars. The blood then carries these tiny nutrients to every single cell in the body, where they serve as food or fuel for the cell. When the sugar is pulled into the cell, it is converted into energy for your body.

One fact that was not understood years ago when I got diabetes was that the carbohydrate we eat turns into glucose (sugar). I remember being told in the past to go ahead and eat what I wanted, as long as it did not have refined sugar added to it. At that time, we did not understand that natural fruits, milks, and starches—in fact, all foods with carbohydrate—turn into glucose or sugar in the blood. Later, as we get into meal planning—notice I did not say "diet"—counting carbohydrates in the food you eat will allow you much more flexibility than people with diabetes had in the past.

Second, the healthy pancreas produces a hormone called glucagon. **Glucagon** acts as a messenger, telling the liver how much sugar to release into the bloodstream. The liver stores sugar in a form we call glycogen. When the glucagon arrives, it tells the liver to release its stored sugar directly into the bloodstream. The liver also converts proteins and other nutrients into sugar as needed. This conversion process is called **gluconeogenesis**. Typically, the liver releases more of this sugar when you have gone a long period without eating, such as when you sleep or fast. Again, the hormone glucagon works with the liver to regulate the sugar level in the bloodstream and, specifically, to protect your body from suffering from too little sugar. If there is not enough sugar in the bloodstream, your organs, especially your brain, cannot be nourished and will not have the energy they need to do their jobs. If this sugar deficiency occurs, you may experience the symptoms of hypoglycemia, or low blood sugar, which we will talk about later.

Third, the pancreas produces and releases **insulin** into the bloodstream. Insulin is the only hormone in the body that can lower the blood sugar level. Blood sugar levels can be raised by various hormones, such as the stress hormones, male or female hormones, and all emotional response hormones. Insulin, however, is the only one that can lower or normalize blood sugar levels. Insulin also functions as a storage hormone, storing fats and other nutrients for later use. In addition, the insulin hormone regulates the breakdown and buildup of protein, used by many structures of the body.

Everyone must have insulin in order to live. Either your body produces some insulin or you must get it from another source. I will explain insulin more fully in a moment.

Working together, the digestive enzymes, the glucagon, and the insulin from the pancreas make a major contribution to the process of converting food into sugar, which the cells turn into energy. They regulate the balance of sugar in the blood. If there is not enough sugar, the pancreas releases the glucagon messenger to tell the liver to release its stored-sugar fuel to raise the blood sugar level. Conversely, if there is too much sugar in the bloodstream, the pancreas releases insulin to help lower the sugar level.

Insulin does not lower the blood sugar level by destroying the sugar or getting rid of it. Insulin simply provides a pathway for the sugar to go out of the bloodstream. After the digestive enzymes have broken down your food into small pieces of sugar, the sugar is then absorbed into the bloodstream. Sugar in the bloodstream does not give us energy, as many people think. The reason we must have some sugar in the bloodstream is because the blood has the ability to circulate that sugar to every single part of the body, specifically to every cell in the body. It is in the cell where sugar is converted to energy, not in the bloodstream. This is also where we get into trouble with diabetes.

There are thousands of cells in the body, each with a specific job to do. Some make up your heart tissue, others create your skin color, and some make up your nerves, so you can feel. And all cells turn sugar into energy to support the organ they are in charge of, as well as for the body in general. Every cell in the body must have sugar in order to do its job and to create energy for the body. However, most cells will not automatically let the sugar in. Think about your house for a minute. Your house has several doors that will allow you to get inside—a front door, back door, garage door, or sliding glass door. If you want to get inside, you normally choose one of these doors to go through. If all these doors are locked, you need a key to unlock them. Once you place the key in the lock, the door will open and you can get inside. It works the same way with the cell. The cell has many doors to let the sugar in, but they are all locked. A body without diabetes readily makes the key to keep the doors open as needed: The key is insulin.

Insulin is critical for your body to use the sugar that comes from the food you eat because it is the only key that allows sugar into the cells. In those of us that have diabetes, either the insulin is not there, there is not enough of it, or the insulin we are making is not effective. Whichever it is, we must find some way to restore enough effective insulin for the body, so that we can process food correctly, have energy, and feel good.

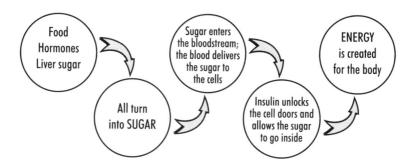

Here's another analogy that sometimes helps. We all know that in order for a car to have energy it has to have gasoline. However, it does not do any good to wash the car in gasoline or to place a can of gasoline in the front seat. For the gasoline to make the car run, the gasoline must be in the fuel tank and get inside the engine. To put gasoline into the car, we use a pump that fits into the opening or door made specifically for gasoline. Once you access that opening and pump the gasoline in, the car can be off and running. It is the very same with all the cells in the body.

It does no good to have the sugar on the outside of the cells; we need it on the inside. So the body uses insulin to open the cell doors to allow the sugar in. Once the sugar is in, the cell converts it into energy, and the cell can do its job. Many people think that diabetes is about avoiding sugar. This is not true. Diabetes is about getting sugar to its correct and final destination. The body needs sugar, just as it needs insulin, in order to thrive. We just need it in a specific place—inside the cells. Now that you know what is supposed to happen, let's look at the reasons sugar does not get inside the cells by discussing the different types of diabetes.

Chapter 3

What type of diabetes do I have or does that even matter?

Over the years I have seen the types of diabetes named and renamed, even though the problems remain the same. Some of the different names are type A, type B, type C, sugar diabetes, diabetes mellitus, adult-onset diabetes, juvenile-onset diabetes, insulin-resistant diabetes, insulin-deficient diabetes, maturity-onset diabetes of the young, borderline, impaired glucose tolerance, insulin dependent diabetes mellitus, non-insulin dependent diabetes mellitus, latent autoimmune diabetes in adults, gestational diabetes, secondary diabetes, type 1, and type 2. It may be helpful to know the type of diabetes you have, but the most important thing is knowing what you need to do to keep your blood sugar in a near-normal range. The type of diabetes you have does not dictate an automatic course of treatment. Your glucose levels determine your treatment.

Regardless of the type of diabetes, good glucose control is critical. High blood sugar levels can damage every part of the body. No matter the type of diabetes, meal planning and exercise are the keys to success. With any type of diabetes, your blood sugar levels can go too high or too low. And regardless of the type or severity of diabetes, it is now recommended that everyone check his or her blood sugars at home. The biggest difference in the types of diabetes may be in the form of medication used to treat it. However, I think it helps to know what might not be working right in your body, because it helps you understand the recommendations for diabetes care. So in the easiest way I know how, I will explain the different factors that may lead to diabetes in its more common forms.

Type 1 Diabetes
(Insulin-dependent or juvenile-onset diabetes)

Type 1 diabetes is typically the result of the destruction of the islet cells located in the pancreas. It is the islet cells' job to produce insulin over the course of your entire life. Your immune system is in charge of getting rid of viruses. Sometimes, when the immune system attempts to destroy a virus, it unfortunately ends up killing the insulin-producing cells as well. We're still not sure exactly why this happens, but we do know that those with type 1 diabetes no longer have the part of the pancreas that generates insulin. This is why people with type 1 diabetes must take insulin injections the rest of their lives.

We don't know what triggers this destructive process. However, we do know the body's immune system plays a part in the destruction, so we call type 1 diabetes an **autoimmune disease**. This means that the person's own immune system has destroyed the insulin-producing cells, known as beta cells. The destruction may come on quickly or slowly. Some people will produce just enough insulin to keep them from developing certain complications for years. (Keep in mind that the pancreas still has working parts, it's just the insulin-producing cells that are being destroyed.)

Type 2 Diabetes
(Non–insulin-dependent, or adult-onset diabetes)

Type 2 diabetes typically occurs in adults over the age of 40 and accounts for 90–95% of all forms of diabetes. The risk for type 2 diabetes increases with age, obesity, lack of physical activity, family history of the disease, previous gestational diabetes, hypertension, and high blood fat levels. The symptoms of type 2 diabetes can be vague, or in the presence of illness, they may be severe. With type 2 diabetes, it is not unusual for complications to develop before you even know you have it. In other words, a complication resulting from the diabetes can be the symptom that actually gets you diagnosed with the disease.

The different types of type 2 diabetes involve multiple errors in the body's metabolic process. Three basic problems are involved and are discussed below. First, type 2 diabetes usually includes decreased insulin production that is not caused by beta cell destruction. Second, the cells have become resistant to insulin. Third, there tends to be an excessive output of glucose by the liver.

Insulin deficiency. The pancreas has cells that are responsible for making insulin. For some reason, in type 2 diabetes, some of these beta cells start slacking off in their duty to produce insulin. The cells are not being destroyed, as in type 1 diabetes, but instead are just not doing an adequate job of producing insulin. Some beta cells are only doing part of their job, others are not doing anything at all, and then some are trying to make up the work for those that are not pulling their load. The bottom line is that the pancreas does not make enough insulin for the body.

Sometimes the amount of insulin is not enough for your body weight. For example, perhaps your pancreas is making enough for a 120-pound person, but you weigh 150 pounds. In this case, you would be deficient in insulin. In some cases weight loss helps, but your pancreas may be able to make enough insulin for only an 80-pound person. The goal, then, is not for you to drop your weight down to 80 pounds. There are other forms of treatment when weight loss is not needed.

There is usually some stored insulin in the pancreas. When the blood sugar begins to rise, this insulin is supposed to be released into the bloodstream, and the liver is supposed to stop releasing its stored glucose. With type 2 diabetes, many people have lost this insulin release to balance the rising blood sugar, and the liver continues to release glucose. Without adequate insulin, proteins, which are responsible for the growth of cells, muscles, and tendons, break down. Thus the body's rebuilding process is hampered. Low insulin levels allow for increased release of glucose from the liver and the breakdown of stored nutrients into sugar. This metabolic problem may get worse, improve, or stay the same.

If a person were deficient in insulin only, then we would try to stimulate the pancreas to work harder and make more insulin. At the same time, using weight management, exercise, and meal planning, we would try to decrease the amount of insulin the body required. The body, however, is usually not just *deficient* in insulin, it may also be *resistant* to insulin.

Cellular resistance. For years we thought diabetes was always a deficiency of insulin. We have now learned that many adults are more likely to be resistant to their own insulin. The simplest way I know to explain insulin resistance is to compare the cells in your body to your house. Recall that you need insulin to unlock cell doors, just as you need keys to unlock your doors at home. Some of your doors may have one lock on them, while others may have an additional dead bolt. It does not matter how many keys you have to the doorknob lock if you do not have any for the dead bolt. If you do not also have at least one dead bolt key, you still cannot get in the house.

Some people with diabetes have dead bolts on their cell doors. Their pancreas may make lots of insulin, but the cell doors are locked and dead bolted, and the insulin cannot get in. Usually the pancreas will try to make extra insulin to open those doors, but the cells can still resist it. Now both sugar and insulin levels in the bloodstream are high. On top of helping sugar get into the cell, insulin has an additional function, which is to promote fat storage. Because of this, those with cellular resistance to insulin are also at risk for excessive or unexplained weight gain.

Excessive liver output of sugar. The liver is also involved with diabetes. The liver has stored glucose to be used in times of stress or emergency as an extra source of fuel. With all forms of type 2 diabetes, the liver releases stored sugar into the bloodstream excessively and inconsistently, resulting in elevated blood sugars even in the absence of food.

Other contributing factors leading to type 2 diabetes may be the increased need for insulin because of obesity, heredity, certain medications, or other illnesses involving the pancreas or immune system, such as pancreatic cancer, pancreatitis, lupus, thyroid problems, and rheumatoid arthritis treated with steroids.

How the different types of diabetes are diagnosed depends on the circumstances at the time of diagnosis. Diabetes in any form is not easily classified. There seem to be grey areas, and sometimes it seems the diagnosis changes, especially in adults. In reality there are probably hundreds of types of diabetes, which is why some people are more prone to complications, whereas others seem to fly by without any. It is also difficult to convince a physician that something is wrong when you look perfectly well. The guidelines for the diagnosis of diabetes include the following glucose levels:

1. Fasting glucose >126

2. Blood sugar >200 two hours after a 75-gram glucose (sugar) intake

3. Random glucose >200 with symptoms

Regardless of the type of diabetes you have, your treatment needs to be individualized. No rules are set in stone, and the rules we do have change relatively frequently as we learn more about diabetes and its treatment. Regrettably, what worked great for you in the beginning may not work forever. And you need to understand that even if you are the same age, sex, weight, and height as your neighbor, your treatment will probably be different. It seems that there are as many ways to manage diabetes as there are people who have diabetes.

QUESTIONS

Why me?

We don't know all the causes of diabetes, but we are pretty sure that heredity and weight play a big part in the development of type 2 diabetes. Heredity affects how much and how long the pancreas will be able to make insulin, and it plays a part in putting the dead bolts on the cell doors, creating insulin resistance. Just because your parents had diabetes does not guarantee you will also get it, but you are more at risk. On the other hand, just because your parents didn't have diabetes does not guarantee you won't get it either. Diabetes sticks to few rules. It chooses without an obvious reason or explanation. We know that increased weight contributes to insulin resistance as well as decreased effectiveness of the insulin you do make. In addition, certain medications or illnesses can make cells more resistant to insulin and place an excessive demand on the pancreas for insulin.

What if I don't have diabetes yet or I'm just borderline?

First of all, you need to understand that you cannot be "just about diabetic." That is like saying you are just about pregnant. Unfortunately, it will take years for old terms like "borderline" to be dropped from the diabetes vocabulary.

If you have been diagnosed with the following, consider yourself to have diabetes:

- Chronic hyperglycemia = diabetes
- Just about diabetic = diabetes
- Borderline diabetes = diabetes or impaired glucose tolerance (IGT)
- Blood sugars that are just a bit too high = diabetes
- Just a touch of sugar = diabetes
- Blood sugars are only high because of your weight = diabetes
- Blood sugars are high because of chronic stress = diabetes

Many physicians try to cushion the blow of diabetes by not calling it what it truly is. They avoid calling diabetes what it is out of the goodness of their hearts and concern for your feelings. But even done in kindness, being told that you "just about have diabetes" can be a disservice to you. If you "just about have diabetes," should you "just about treat it"? Many patients I have worked with feel as if they have failed because they were only borderline for years, yet now they have full-blown diabetes. The strange thing about this is that they already have complications of diabetes—even though they have supposedly not had diabetes.

It is not that I want everyone scared to death when their blood sugar is just a bit elevated. What I want you to know is that now is the time to take action and start treatment. By taking steps early in the management of meal plans, exercise, and blood checking, you may be able to keep your diabetes in control and require no medication for years. It does not serve you well to wait until blood sugars have been high for a while and complications have started, and then try to make lifestyle changes.

There is no benefit to not knowing the full story. The sooner you know you have diabetes, the sooner you can do something about it. Diabetes undiagnosed is diabetes untreated. And diabetes that goes untreated has serious consequences.

Sometimes I think it would be easier to diagnose diabetes by a diabetes level classification system. The levels would have to do solely with what is required for management rather than what is causing the diabetes. Diagnosis by what causes the diabetes does not always tell us what we need to do to manage it. My diagnostic system would work something like Table 3-1.

TABLE 3-1. DIABETES LEVELS AND TREATMENTS

PRE DIABETES	meal planning, exercise, weight loss, yearly blood glucose test at your doctor's office
LEVEL ONE DIABETES	meal planning, exercise, and blood checking are needed for management
LEVEL TWO DIABETES	meal planning, exercise, blood checking, and oral medications are needed for management
LEVEL THREE DIABETES	meal planning, exercise, blood checking, and oral and occasional insulin use are needed for management
LEVEL FOUR DIABETES	meal planning, exercise, blood checking, and insulin injections are needed for management

Diabetes is serious, no matter the degree or level or classification. Now is the time to do something about it—not later when there are complications.

If I lose a bunch of weight, can I lose my diabetes?

I wish weight loss were a cure for diabetes—it isn't—but it is an effective treatment. By losing weight you may lose the need for medication, but the diabetes is still there. Your blood sugar levels may stay in range just by your following meal plans and exercising. However, if you regain the weight or stop watching what you eat, the need for medication will likely return. We cannot cure diabetes yet, but we can manage it very well. Let this be your goal.

If there's so much sugar in me, why don't I have any energy?

(Short-term complications of high glucose levels)

Our bodies are amazing machines. When one part of it is not working, another part kicks in and works harder to try and compensate. For example, if the right lung has been damaged or removed, the left lung compensates by taking in more air. If your left eye is lazy, your right eye learns to focus better. When blood sugar levels go up, the body has ways to compensate as well. The body's attempt to compensate is where some of the symptoms come in. Let us look at the more common symptoms of diabetes and why they occur.

Symptoms of Diabetes

Increased thirst and increased urination—which came first? I remember as a child going on a picnic where we forgot to bring a drink. My thirst was so severe I panicked at the thought of not having anything to drink. Several times during that short period of time I drank out of a mud puddle because I didn't think I would make it otherwise. When we got home I remember drinking 10 or 11 full glasses of water all at once. I could hear the water sloshing around in my stomach, and I felt waterlogged—but I was still craving water.

I call it the chicken or the egg question. Which came first, increased urination or increased thirst. I believe the problem starts with the increased urination. The kidneys have the job of being filters for the blood. They decide what is good or bad, what should stay in the bloodstream or be kicked out as waste in the form of urine. An easy way to understand the job of a kidney is to compare it to a dishwasher. As the dishwasher runs its cycle, it cleans the waste off the dishes, which then results in clean dishes that you can use again. Your kidneys do the same thing. When the blood sugar level rises above 180mg/dl, the kidneys know there is too much sugar in the blood. The kidneys help by filtering the excess sugar out into the urine. In order for the sugar to get out, however, it has to be dissolved in water so it can be passed out in the urine. So the more sugar the kidney needs to filter out, the more water in the form of urine we put out as well.

Naturally, to compensate for the loss of water, your thirst centers are going to make you thirsty in an attempt to get you to drink to replace the water you have lost and to prevent dehydration. Thus begins a vicious cycle of drinking and urinating. Unfortunately, the kidneys cannot filter out all the excess sugar in your body, so this process will continue as long as the blood sugars are elevated.

Several imbalances occur when you have this kind of excessive urination—dehydration, weight loss, and electrolyte imbalances, to name a few. Dehydration occurs from the loss of fluid and the increased need for it. Weight loss comes from the sugar and calories that are being urinated out. This calorie loss can also lead to increased hunger. Electrolyte imbalances occur because excessive amounts of sodium, potassium, magnesium, calcium, and chloride are passed along with the urine.

Dry, itchy skin; dry mouth. This is due to the dehydration and chemical imbalances caused by excessive urination. The mouth is a mucous membrane, and any time blood sugars are high, the mucous membranes of the body will be sugar coated, and hence make the mouth sticky and dry, and sometimes sweet or metallic tasting.

Obvious, unexplainable weight gain or loss. Weight loss is usually something adults celebrate, rather than worry about. We all hope for the day when the weight will come off without us having to do anything to promote it. However, the weight loss associated with undiagnosed diabetes is an unhealthy, rapid weight loss, and the weight usually returns when glucose control is improved. The weight loss may be due to dehydration, calories passed in the urine, or ketone production (which will be discussed later). On the other hand, weight gain may be caused by resistance of the cells to insulin, so your body produces more insulin. Excessive amounts of insulin promote fat storage. In addition, a lack of energy can lead to less activity, which can also cause weight gain. Obesity may be one of the triggers that bring on type 2 diabetes.

Vision change. Any time the blood sugar is elevated, the mucous membranes of the body will have sugar on them. Well, the eye is another mucous membrane. As sugar builds up on the lens, the lens becomes swollen, or thicker and stiff. The lens of your eye should be thin and flexible so it can adjust to whatever you are looking at. When the lens is swollen or stiff, it cannot adjust correctly and vision becomes blurry. Some days, vision will be better, some days worse. (Occasionally, if patients actually need a thicker lens, their vision improves with the onset of diabetes.) These vision changes are temporary, however. Once blood sugars have returned to normal for one or two months, the blurriness will clear up, unless there is a need for corrective lenses.

Frequent infections. Frequent infections, such as yeast, urinary, sinus, wound, kidney, or skin sores are common prior to the diagnosis of diabetes, because blood sugar levels are higher than they should be. Several factors contribute to increased infections. White blood cells, which help to defend the body from infection, have more difficulty finding the bacteria. When the white blood cells do find the bacteria, they have less ability to destroy them. Finally, bacteria cells thrive in the presence of sugar.

Let's compare the white blood cells to a car on a highway. If you are driving into a big city between 2:00 and 3:00 a.m., there are fewer cars on the freeway, so you can get to your destination faster. However, during rush hour traffic, you stop and go, speed up and slow down, and it takes much longer. It works the same way with the white blood cells. When blood sugar levels are high, the blood is thicker and stickier, and the white blood cells have difficulty finding their way to the infected site to fight the bacteria. When the white blood cells finally do find the bacteria, they are so exhausted from fighting all the traffic that they have only half their ability to destroy the bacteria. And finally, bacteria cells need sugar in order to grow and reproduce. If your blood sugar levels are high, the bacteria cells are in hog heaven.

No energy. Some of the most common complaints I hear from patients are that they get tired after eating, can't stay awake when sitting still, and need to nap constantly—yet they never feel rested. We've always been told that sugar gives us energy, but this is true only when sugar is in the correct place. Remember that in order for sugar in the blood to give us energy, it first has to be delivered to every cell in the body. Once the sugar is in the cell, the energy can be tapped. But if sugar is high in the blood, the cells are not getting their share, so they can't create energy for the body. As a word of caution, don't let diabetes be a scapegoat; look into your habits and patterns. Fatigue could be caused by something else—it could by depression, thyroid disorders, or other medications you are taking.

Muscle cramps. Patients frequently tell me that they experience charley horses, muscle aches, leg pains, and cramping muscles. These symptoms may be the result of an electrolyte imbalance caused by the increased urination and high blood sugars. Sodium, potassium, and chloride help keep muscles, including the heart muscle, contracting and relaxing correctly. When these electrolytes are out of balance, muscles tend to cramp or ache more, and the heart may beat irregularly. Many people treat these symptoms by adding additional sources of electrolytes to their diet, such as bananas, milk, and fruits. These foods may temporarily ease the cramps, but they do not treat the underlying cause. Lowering blood sugar levels will prevent the frequent urination and loss of electrolytes.

High blood pressure, headaches. Atherosclerosis (hardening of the arteries caused by a buildup of plaque), increased thickness of the blood, and the heart having to work harder to pump the thick, sticky blood all over the body can lead to high blood pressure. Typically, hardening of the arteries is caused by excess plaque or cholesterol, but high blood sugars add an extra coat of sugar to the arteries' walls.

High blood pressure can cause headaches, migraines, and dizziness. However, headaches can also be caused by visual disturbances associated with high blood sugars, by brain cells saturated with sugar, and by decreased circulation to the small vessels of the brain. And sometimes we do not know the cause.

Sexual dysfunction. Sexual dysfunction can occur in both men and women. When blood sugars are high, the nerves in the body are damaged and cannot respond, relay, or receive messages from the brain correctly. As a result, men may experience impotence or erectile dysfunction. Women may have genital pain, inadequate lubrication, and an inability to have an orgasm. However, remember that these sexual problems can also be caused by injury, emotional problems, or medications.

Decreased ability to concentrate. I recall a medical student who was unaware he was developing diabetes. He was a top-of-the-class student, had excellent grades, and had big plans in the medical field. As his blood sugars crept up, he found it harder to concentrate and remember the material, and he began to think something was wrong with him. But once his diabetes was diagnosed and his blood sugar levels returned to normal, so did his ability to process and concentrate.

Of all the cells in the body, the ones that need sugar the most are the brain cells. This is because our brain has some control of every single function of the body. To protect this amazing organ from being deprived of nutrition, the brain cells do not require insulin to let the sugar in. So when blood sugar levels are high, the brain is being saturated with sugar. With all this excess sugar, the brain cannot work properly; it needs balance.

Numbness or tingling in feet or fingers. Numbness in the feet or fingers often indicates that blood sugar levels have been elevated for some time, even for years. The numbness may be the result of nerves damaged by high blood sugars or poor nutrition, and it can lead to an inability to interpret tactile information correctly. This nerve damage, called *neuropathy*, may occur anywhere in the body, but it is most common in the feet and fingers at diagnosis.

No obvious symptoms. There are several reasons the symptoms of diabetes are sometimes not recognized. First, most adults in the early stages of diabetes are still making some insulin, just not enough, so the symptoms are mild. A body can stay at this stage for years. Second, some symptoms of diabetes resemble those that occur during pregnancy, for example, as well as in depression, stress, or other illnesses. And third, adults can blame many of the symptoms on age or age-related treatments. Increased urination may be caused by water pills, prostate problems, or urinary tract infections—or because you are trying to drink the recommended eight glasses of water a day. Increased thirst may be explained away because you do not drink enough water or because you are taking water pills. Cramps may be attributed to poor eating habits. Vision changes are associated with aging. And weight gain may be blamed on lack of exercise. Adults rarely see weight loss as a symptom that something might be wrong.

Depression and mood swings. Consider the flip side of "no obvious symptoms." Let's say you are getting up five or six times a night to go to the bathroom, you frequently trip on something because your vision is blurry, and before getting back into bed you get a drink of water because your mouth is so dry. Then when you are finally comfortable in bed you have a charley horse that seems to last forever. And when you recover from that you have to go to the bathroom again. Your skin is dry and itchy. Food, which is supposed to give you energy, doesn't. Even if you do get to stay in bed, you do not feel rested.

How well can a person feel going through this night after night, week after week, sometimes for months on end? These bothersome symptoms lead to sleeplessness and physical, mental, and emotional exhaustion. It is a cycle that feeds itself. Lack of sleep leads to tiredness, which leads to inability to function during the day, which causes unhappiness at work and poor coping skills. The more you rest, the worse you feel and the higher your glucose levels rise. Depression and mood swings are understandable. Not only do the symptoms interfere with your life, but they can also cause chemical imbalances, which lead to mood swings, tiredness, and depression as well. (Later I will address depression associated with chronic illness.)

At this point we know what is supposed to be happening, what is not happening and why, and what the symptoms are telling us. Now what are we going to do about it? There are several corner-stones of diabetes management for all types of diabetes:

- meal planning

- blood glucose checking

- exercise, medication, and

- chronic disease management.

Chapter 5

Why should I check my blood sugar? I thought only people on insulin had to do that.

Before we had the use of blood glucose meters, we checked the urine for sugar. We did not know at the time—nor could we do anything else—how inaccurate urine testing for sugar was. Urine results may be influenced by how much fluid you've had to drink, the last time you went to the bathroom, kidney function, and other drugs you may be taking. Urine sugar results were also easy to manipulate. The urine sugar level may reflect a blood sugar level of eight or more hours prior to the test. Another thing to take note of is that sugar does not typically show up in the urine until the blood sugar level is above 180 mg/dl. That is too late. This means you could have blood sugars running 140–180 mg/dl all the time, but sugar never shows up in your urine. This situation is not good. Finally in the late 1970s, a much more accurate way to check blood sugar levels was created.

Checking Blood Sugar Levels

Blood glucose checking at home is the most accurate tool we have to determine if our diabetes management efforts are working.

Checking your blood sugar gives you immediate information on the effects of your food choices, exercise, and medication. It also helps to eliminate some of the guesswork when you are not feeling just right and you are wondering, "Is it my diabetes or something else?" Many patients tell me that they can just tell if their blood sugar is too high or too low. The problem with this is that it is not reliable. Symptoms can fool you, especially the longer you have diabetes. But we also do not want patients running high enough or low enough to feel it. Blood sugars can creep up very slowly, and you still feel perfectly fine. You may also feel the same when you are running 70–140 mg/dl as you do 60–250 mg/dl. The first is okay, the second is not.

The bottom line: Blood monitoring at home is the only way you and your health care professionals can safely and knowledgeably adjust your diabetes medications. You may have times of the day when you tend to run higher or lower, times when you need more medication and times when you need less. If medications are added before you know these patterns, they can actually make you feel worse rather than better. Most medication mismanagement problems can be avoided with blood sugar monitoring. Home glucose checking also reassures you that exercising and meal planning do make a difference.

What should blood sugar levels be? Ideally, blood glucose levels should be as close to normal as possible, that is, 80–130 mg/dl. However, this is not always possible, nor is it always safe. Keeping blood sugar close to normal means that we will flirt with hypoglycemia or low blood sugar. This is not safe for young children, who need a constant amount of glucose for normal brain development, or for those who cannot recognize the symptoms of hypoglycemia or do not know how to self-treat. In the elderly, hypoglycemia can cause falls or confusion and can make the person more prone to a stroke. If a person does not recognize symptoms of hypoglycemia or is not able to treat hypoglycemia independently for any reason, glucose goals may need to be raised to avoid problems.

All that aside, the American Diabetes Association and research studies recommend plasma glucose goals that run 90–130 mg/dl before meals and less than 180 two hours after eating. There are a few additional things to know.

Aim for a range. Do not aim for a specific number, aim for a blood sugar range. You will succeed more often. Even people without diabetes do not have blood sugars that stay the same. With blood sugar levels changing every one or two minutes, you can drive yourself crazy limiting what your results can be. Aiming for a specific number will simply lead to frustration.

Check frequently. Because glucose levels change constantly, one check a week or a month does not give enough information to make any educated adjustments in your treatment plan.

Remember that blood sugars are neither good nor bad. The number that shows up on your meter is a not a judgment of your worth or value as a person. Glucose levels give information and direction on what to do next. They tell us if treatment plans are working, or where and when they need to be changed. Do your best not to judge yourself from these numbers. Then you will find it easier to check more often with less resentment.

How often and when should I check? The answer to this depends on the type of diabetes you have and the medications being used. If you are using insulin, at least four blood checks a day, prior to meals, are needed for good, safe management. The more often you check, the more accurate you can be in insulin adjustments. When you take pills to manage diabetes, two to four checks a day, before meals, are most helpful. By breaking the day into time frames, you can see what your blood sugar does over a 24-hour period. When checking twice a day, checks before breakfast and dinner one day, rotated with checks before lunch and at bedtime the next day, still give you adequate information needed for safe adjustments. For patients on meal planning and exercise management only, one to two checks daily is recommended.

If your physician asks you to check blood sugars after a meal, you need to check what your blood sugar is before eating as well. Otherwise you will know if the blood sugar is high, but you will not know if it is because of the food you just ate or if it was high prior to eating. Once blood sugars have come into range, do not stop checking. Blood sugars can climb very slowly without warnings. If you cut back to checking several times a week, rotate the times you check and go back to more frequent checking if your numbers begin to elevate.

How to read blood sugar records: Be a detective. Reading blood sugar levels is like reading a mystery or playing detective. You need to pay attention to details and patterns, come up with theories and questions, and then review the records again to find a solution. Figuring out what blood sugars mean can be tricky. But you are the detective with the best insight. When looking at the data you have kept, look for a pattern at a specific time of day. Some people find it easy to see patterns if they highlight or circle blood sugars that are either in or out of range. If you do this, I recommend highlighting the blood sugars that are in range. It seems kind of petty, but it helps to focus on the positive instead of the negative. When you have found a way to look at your data, ask this question: Is there a time of day when you typically run high or low? Do you typically wake up high, or do you go higher throughout the day? Finding patterns like this helps you to know the best time to give medications or what part of the day you need to adjust medication or meal planning. This is made easier by keeping a blood glucose diary or record book that breaks your day into breakfast, lunch, dinner, and bedtime.

Knowing that a blood sugar goal is usually between 80–130 and 80–140 acceptably, let us look at the following blood sugars and see what patterns we find. Blood sugars were checked before breakfast, lunch, snack, dinner, and at bedtime.

EXAMPLE 1

What patterns do you see? (Blood sugars are checked before meals.)

	B	L	Sn	D	B	Comments
MON	139	210		245	316	
TUE	156	219		268	328	
WED	101	234		246	317	
THU	137	214		281	345	
FRI	138	213		219	331	

Patterns

1. The lowest blood sugars of the day are the fasting or waking blood sugars.
2. The highest blood sugars are at bedtime.
3. The blood sugars tend to rise across the day.

Questions we could ask

1. Has meal planning or any diabetes medication been started? If not, it's time.

EXAMPLE 2

What patterns do you see? (Blood sugars are checked before meals.)

	B	L	Sn	D	B	Comments
MON	87	110		221	127	
TUE	94	128		215	113	
WED	83	132		234	137	
THU	87	112		210	98	
FRI	89	110		214	101	

Patterns

1. Blood sugars are in the desired range throughout the day except at dinner (evening meal).

Questions we could ask

1. What is this person having for lunch? Maybe he needs to eat smaller servings.

2. Is this person having a snack in the afternoon? Maybe the snack needs to be changed from a sandwich and chips to a half sandwich and a diet drink.

3. Could this person check blood sugars in the afternoon? This would help identify whether it was the lunch or the snack that raises the dinnertime blood sugar.

EXAMPLE 3

What patterns do you see? (Blood sugars are checked before meals.)

	B	L	Sn	D	B	Comments
MON	187	100		101	92	
TUE	210	123		97	101	
WED	174	132		116	89	
THU	168	113		126	94	
FRI	181	110		129	98	

Patterns

1. Fasting blood sugar levels are consistently above desired range.

2. Nighttime blood sugar levels are in range—and the lowest of the day.

Questions we could ask

1. Is the person eating during the night, possibly causing a higher morning reading? If so, decreasing nighttime snacking might help.

2. Is the person treating hypoglycemia during the night, causing higher fasting levels? If this is true, decreasing the nighttime medication might help.

3. When does this person last eat? Perhaps the last meal of the day is at 4:30 p.m. and the high waking blood sugars are the result of the liver kicking in to provide sugar for the body. In this case, adding a snack with protein before bed might decrease the need for the liver to release stored sugar.

EXAMPLE 4

What patterns do you see? (Blood sugars are checked before meals.)

	B	L	Sn	D	B	Comments
MON	98	112		97	83	
TUE	87	101		87	199	birthday party 7 p.m.
WED	89	111		93	96	
THU	92	113		94	90	
FRI	87	234*	212	167	123	flat tire on way to work

Patterns

1. Blood sugar levels appear well managed except on special occasions.

Questions we could ask

1. Does this person know how to adjust meal plans for special foods or occasions? If not, he or she needs to learn.

2. Does this person have a plan for high-stress days or events? He should ask his diabetes educator for help to create a plan.

FINAL EXAMPLE

What patterns do you see? (Blood sugars are checked before meals.)

	B	L	Sn	D	B	Comments
MON	178	56		119	431	
TUE	216	417		52	179	
WED	300	299		321	46	
THU	101	376		123	234	
FRI	194	65		456	72	

Patterns

1. There is no pattern; at each time of day there are some normal, high, and low glucose levels.

Questions we could ask

1. Is this person following a meal plan? When we see numbers like this, the first area to address is meal planning. Nothing will have a greater effect on the blood sugar than consistent mealtimes and amounts of food.

Blood Glucose Meters

Checking your blood sugars at home has become relatively simple. You can choose from about thirty different machines, each having features you may or may not need or want. Most of the machines require a strip of some sort to apply a drop of blood to. Each strip can be used only once, so expense will be something to consider when picking a machine. I feel pretty safe to say that most of the machines are given to you for free by the different manufacturers because they know that if you have their machine, you will have to use their strips. Each machine should also come with some type of blood-letting device to prick the finger or arm or leg, and these are interchangeable between machines. It does not matter which device you use to get the blood; it is the size of the drop of blood that counts. Try several different devices to see if you feel more comfortable with one. Ask your diabetes nurse educator for recommendations.

A note on all meters—they are not perfect. Blood glucose meters are the best tool we have to measure the management of your diabetes, but that does not mean they can't fail or won't misread. They are machines that require you to be correct in coding, timing, the size of blood drop, and in use of the correct type of strip. In addition, meters and strips may have been exposed to extremes of heat and cold, splashing and banging, or dropped in water, all of which will affect the accuracy. Keep in mind there can always be manufacture error as well. Most machines will give a lower reading than the lab. Get to know your meter. Try using one or two meters consistently. Since not all meters read the same, you will drive yourself crazy comparing blood sugars on more than two different meters at the same time. If your machine gives you a reading you feel is incorrect, be sure your fingers are clean and dry and that you have a fresh, hanging drop of blood. You will need to recalibrate your meter occasionally using a test solution from the manufacturer.

Tips for Increasing Meter-Reading Accuracy

- Be sure your fingers are clean and dry.

- Have a fresh, hanging drop of blood.

- Avoid double dipping or applying blood twice to the test strip.

- Make sure that your strips have not expired.

- Double-check the strip code number.

- If you question your result, perform another test on the same machine, being as precise as possible in your technique.

- Call the meter manufacture if you believe the meter is inaccurate. All meters have a toll-free telephone number for troubleshooting 24 hours a day.

Monitoring Tricks

- Warm your hands.

- Poke the corner of your fingers, not the tip or midline.

- Milk the finger prior to and after poking it.

- Wrap an elastic band around your finger so that the blood is forced to the tip, then poke the finger. Be careful—sometimes it squirts.

- Use a pricking device that allows you to adjust the depth of the poke.

- Instead of squeezing the tip of your finger, squeeze from the palm toward the tip of the finger to trap the blood there.

- Try a meter that takes blood from another site, such as an arm or leg.

Take Note

- Alcohol can change the chemical reaction on the test strip. If you want to use it, be sure that the alcohol has dried before you poke the finger.

- Dirt, juice, sweat, or any chemical can change the reaction on the test strip. For the most accurate results, be sure you have clean hands and use the same technique each time you test.

- Extremes in temperature can change the result on the test strip.

- Home glucose testing is not cheap. If you need to check four times a day, you can cut back on the cost by rotating the times you check. For example, one day check at breakfast and dinner, then the next day check at lunch and bedtime. You will still get the results you need, just not as quickly.

QUESTIONS

My physician told me not to worry about checking my blood sugars at home. He'd just run an A1C test every three months. What is an A1C test, and is that recommendation acceptable?

Physicians may say this to ease the inconvenience of poking your finger every day, but it still leaves you with a lot of guesswork when it comes to adjusting medications. An A1C test is a blood test that tells what your overall average blood sugar has been for the past two to three months. This test takes into account the good days and the bad, 24 hours a day, for this full 90-day time period, not just the checks you might have done on your meter. For those who cannot or will not check, an A1C test gives some information on their overall control. But it is a much more effective tool if used in combination with the home blood monitoring, which is more accurate in identifying patterns.

A desired level for an A1C for adults is 7.0 or less (whichever is the upper limit of normal for your doctor's laboratory). This works out to be an average blood sugar of about 140 mg/dl. The graph below (Table 5-1) will give you an idea of how an A1C level is related to blood sugar levels. The lab you use may have a different scale, so be sure to find out what normal is on its scale.

TABLE 5-1. A1C AND BLOOD SUGAR LEVELS

A1C Value		Blood Sugar Value
14	→	>360
13	→	330
12	→	300
11	→	270
10	→	240
9	→	210
8	→	180
7	→	140
6	→	120
5	→	90

Knowing what you do about blood monitoring and looking for patterns, how would you answer the question "Is it okay to do only A1C tests?" Let's say you had a result of 9.0, which would indicate a blood sugar average of 210 mg/dl. Is this acceptable? We know it is not, so the next question is, "Where do we add or adjust medications?" We do not know. The best we can do is guess. Without record keeping at home, we do not know if you are always high at a specific time of day, or if you are high all the time. What exactly is the problem with only doing an A1C test every three months? Not enough data. I look at an A1C test like a compass. It tells us which direction we are heading and whether we are on or off course. If we are off course, the individual daily blood checks will tell us how to get back on course, much like a trail of bread crumbs leads us out of the forest. For the best management, use blood sugar checks daily combined with an A1C test every three months.

What medications are used to treat diabetes?

Medications can be as tricky to figure out as blood sugars are. I have found that an easy way to understand diabetes medications is to compare them to pain medications. Think about these different situations related to a severe injury.

Let us say you are at home with a badly broken leg and someone stops by once a day to give you a pain pill. If you can only have one pain pill a day, how long must that painkiller last? Obviously, it had better last at least 24 hours. If you are taking only one pill a day to manage your diabetes, it also needs to last 24 hours. Your body hurts when your diabetes medication wears off because blood sugars go high, just as your leg hurts when the pain medication wears off. Even if you only need meal planning and exercise, they need to work for 24 hours as well.

Now let's say that you can have a pain pill as often as you need it. You have found that one pill lasts about three and a half hours. Is it better to wait until that pill has completely worn off and the pain has returned before you take another one, or should you take your next pill before the first one wears off? If you have been in pain before, you know that it is a good idea to take your next pain pill before the first one has completely worn off. Otherwise, the pain gets out of control and takes longer to get back under control. Your blood sugars work the same way. If you notice that your blood sugars are always high at a certain time of day, you will want to add medication or exercise before that time so that the blood sugar does not have a chance to rise. High blood sugars take longer to come back down and sometimes take more medication, too. We also do not want to play "catch-up" all the time, waiting for levels to go up and then treating them. You will feel better and your body will function better if you prevent the highs whenever possible, rather than just treating them after they occur.

It has been a week since you broke your leg, and as long as you are flat in bed, one pain pill a day works well to control your pain. Tomorrow, however, you are getting up for physical therapy for the first time. Do you think the one pain pill will be enough tomorrow? The first day up can be difficult, and your pain may not be as well controlled. Once again, it works the same with your blood sugars. If you follow a meal plan every day but Saturday, your blood sugars will not be as well controlled on Saturday as they are the rest of the week. This does not mean that you have to eat the exact same thing every day. But consistency in timing and amount does make a difference in how well your blood sugar stays balanced.

And finally, your next-door neighbor broke the same leg on the same day you did. Your neighbor, unlike you, has been able to get along fine with one pain pill a day, even with physical therapy. We can compare this to diabetes, because people with similar circumstances will not require the same medication or routine that you do, even if you weigh the same, eat the same, exercise the same, and are the same age. Everybody is different, and your blood sugar levels will let you know how much and what dose of diabetes medication you need.

Before we go any further, let us make one thing clear. Needing medication to manage your diabetes is **not a sign of failure** on your part. You can eat perfectly, exercise perfectly, lose weight as you were instructed—and you may still need medication. Even when you have done all you can do, your body, your pancreas, and your blood sugar levels have the final say on whether or not medication is needed. Understand that the efforts you do make will reduce the need for medications and help the medication you are taking be more effective. So your efforts are worthwhile. Also, the best diabetes medication cannot control blood sugars without meal planning. You can out-eat any medication.

Diabetes Pills

There are several types of pills for diabetes. These pills are not insulin; as a matter a fact, they are effective only if your body is still making some insulin. To understand what the pills do, let's break the pills into two groups: insulin stimulants and insulin sensitizers (Table 6-1).

If you have a pancreas that is not producing enough insulin for your needs, you may need a pill that will stimulate your pancreas to work harder. If you already have tons of insulin and it just is not doing any good or the cells are resisting it, you need a pill that will decrease the resistance and make you more sensitive to your own insulin.

Once again, compare these medications to pain medications, except this time we are using a morphine drip to control pain. The drip gives a small amount of pain medication continuously to take the edge off. If the pain becomes worse or you are getting up to have physical therapy, you can hit a button that will release extra pain medication. The sensitizers work like the morphine drip. They decrease the resistance of the cells and help your own insulin work better throughout the day. Insulin stimulants can give you an extra boost of insulin when needed.

An additional category of drugs are called **alpha-glucosidase inhibitors.** These drugs (Precose and Glyset) decrease the absorption of carbohydrate in the small intestine. This results in a lower after-meal blood sugar. Side effects include upset stomach and gas, which may be the reason they are not as commonly used as some of the other drugs.

Medications are prescribed when blood sugars will not stay in the desired ranges with exercise and meal planning alone, or if they are quite high to begin with. Your physician may prescribe insulin sensitizers, insulin stimulants, or both. The challenge with medications is that there is no precise way to determine which drug a perrson needs or the right dose. Information such as your weight and glucose records will help health care professionals make an educated guess. Beyond that, prescribing is done by trial and error.

TABLE 6-1. DIABETES PILLS

INSULIN STIMULANTS

Action

1) Decrease cells' resistance

2) Decrease the liver's release of stored glucose

3) Stimulate the pancreas to make and release more insulin

Names
Amaryl (glimepiride)
Glucotrol, Glucotrol XL (glipizide)
Diabeta, Glynase, Micronase, PresTab (glyburide)
Orinase (tolbutamide)
Tolinase (tolazamide)
Prandin (repaglinide)
Starlix (nateglinide)

The difference between these medications is how long they last. Amaryl and Glucotrol are supposed to last up to 24 hours. The drugs listed next, from Diabeta to Tolinase, are usually taken twice a day. Prandin and Starlix last only 1 1/2 to 2 hours.

INSULIN SENSITIZERS

Action

1) Decrease the cells' resistance to insulin

2) Decrease the liver's release of stored glucose

3) Does *not* stimulate the pancreas to make or release insulin

Names
Actos (pioglitazone)
Avandia (rosiglitazone)
Glucophage, **Glucophage XR** (metformin)
Glucovance (metformin + glyburide)

Patients on metformin need to have frequent liver function tests and also need to have healthy kidneys.

Once a medication is added, we watch the blood sugar levels to see if we need to increase or decrease the amount, or to try something else. It is critical that you know the effects of your medication on your blood sugar.

Metformin should not be taken if you have congestive heart failure. Nor should you take metformin if you have kidney disease or dysfunction. Insulin, which is covered later in this chapter, is added when the pills in different combination do not control blood sugars or when pills cannot be taken for some reason.

Let us look at some blood sugar records and see how medication could be used.

EXAMPLE 1

	B	L	Sn	D	B	Comments
MON	139	210		245	316	
TUE	156	219		268	328	
WED	101	234		246	317	
THU	137	214		281	345	
FRI	138	213		219	331	

Medication Needs for Example 1

Because the blood sugars get higher across the day every day, it would be appropriate to start a medication with breakfast. This dose would be increased every couple of weeks until blood sugars return to the desired range. If lowering the glucose levels across the day does not also bring down the waking level, then you could add another medication at dinner or bedtime.

EXAMPLE 2

	B	L	Sn	D	B	Comments
MON	87	110		221	127	
TUE	94	128		215	113	
WED	83	132		234	137	
THU	87	112		210	98	
FRI	89	110		214	101	

Medication Needs for Example 2

Since blood sugars are only high at dinner, before adding medication we might want to try adding exercise in the afternoon or after lunch, or we could decrease the serving size of lunch or snack to see if this would help. If these techniques do not help, then a short-lasting medication such as Prandin could be added with lunch or snack depending on which one is raising the blood sugar.

EXAMPLE 3

	B	L	Sn	D	B	Comments
MON	187	100		101	92	
TUE	210	123		97	101	
WED	174	132		116	89	
THU	168	113		126	94	
FRI	181	110		129	98	

Medication Needs for Example 3

Blood sugar levels that are high only on waking is a common problem that is often mistreated. Assuming that the cause is the liver kicking out sugar during the night, the most appropriate time for medication would be bedtime. Remember that we want to prevent the high blood sugar, not treat it after it's already high. With blood sugars in range at bedtime, it would not be safe to add medication then unless we had this blood sugar history to look at, which shows a consistent rise in blood sugar overnight. Another frequent problem is that blood monitoring is only being done occasionally in the morning—such as a fasting blood sugar at your physician's office. When these levels are high, the physician assumes that blood sugars are high all the time. If medication is added in the morning, what is it going to do to the blood sugars that are already in range? It will drop them too low. And you have to eat all day to treat the low, which defeats your weight-loss plan, and blood sugars get worse.

All this because the medication wasn't matched up with the blood sugar patterns. Can you see how important these records are?

EXAMPLE 4

	B	L	Sn	D	B	Comments
MON	98	112		97	83	
TUE	87	101		87	199	birthday party 7 p.m.
WED	89	111		93	96	
THU	92	113		94	90	
FRI	87	234*	212	167	123	flat tire on way to work

Medication Needs for Example 4

Because blood sugars are in range unless there is stress, no medication change is needed here. However, you could add exercise to compensate for stress or additional eating, or ask for ideas of how to adjust your meal plan for special occasions.

EXAMPLE 5: THE IMPORTANCE OF RECORD KEEPING

	B	L	Sn	D	B	Comments
MON	78	56		91	43	
TUE	21	41		52	17	
WED	30	29		32	46	
THU	71	37		53	64	
FRI	44	65		356	52	

Medication Needs for Example 5

This patient is on insulin injections, is having severe hypoglycemia, and is going to her physician for help in changing the insulin dose. On her way, she runs over a cat, which upsets her, and then she was speeding because she was late and got a speeding ticket. By the time she got to the doctor's office, her blood sugar was 356 from stress, and she had no records for her physician to look at.

Noted patterns: Extremely low blood sugars across the day, **except once.**

Questions we could ask:

If blood sugar that high (356 mg/dl) is the only one the physician sees, the only assumption he or she could make is that blood sugars are running too high. If the physician wants to increase the insulin dose, what will happen? This person is in trouble—she already has too much insulin on board.

This is an extreme example, but it does happen. More commonly we see the opposite situation. The blood sugar levels of individuals typically run high, but on the day they see their physician, they do not eat all day, so their blood sugar is lower than usual. The blood sugar at the office is normal, and no adjustments in medication are made. Who is this helping? No one. Without records, the physician can only guess what to do with the medications. Give your physician the help he or she needs. Always bring your records to your appointments and invite your health care professional to study them.

Most of the pills used to treat diabetes can be taken with a meal. However, for Prandin to be effective, you need to take it before eating. If you forget your pill, usually you can take it as soon as you remember. It is not recommended that you double up a dose. If it is close to the time when you would be taking the next pill, you are better off getting back on track with your next dose.

If your blood sugar levels have been high for a long time, once they come down, you may not need as much medication to keep them down. In the beginning you have thick, sugar-coated cells, kind of like a frosted donut. You need medication to handle the food you eat now, but also for all the leftover sugar-coated cells in your system. Once you get rid of some of the leftovers, you may need less medication to take care of the food you eat.

Insulin

I hear many adults say, "I wish I was on insulin so I could eat whatever I want." This kind of thinking is dangerous. With insulin, you need to be more careful with your diet: You cannot skip meals, you need to check blood sugars more often, and your risk for hypoglycemia is greater. However, when you need insulin, don't avoid it, because nothing else can take its place. And nothing else will help you feel better.

Insulin is used when the pills are not effective or, as in pregnancy, they cannot be used to treat diabetes. Just like the pills for diabetes, insulin also opens cell doors. The types of insulin are different in how fast and how long they work. Some insulins are fast acting; they kick in within 10–30 minutes after taking them, but they do not last very long. Other insulins are long acting—they last for 12–24 hours, but it may take 4–6 hours for them to start working (Table 6-2). You will see a fast-acting insulin combined with a long-acting insulin to provide coverage for a 24-hour period. However, insulin can be used in dozens of different combinations to accommodate different lifestyles and to allow you to be more flexible. I will show you the two most common combinations.

TABLE 6-2. COMMON INSULIN NAMES AND DURATIONS

Humalog and Novolog	fast-acting insulin
Regular	short-acting insulin
NPH	intermediate-acting insulin
Lente	intermediate-acting insulin
Ultralente	long-lasting insulin
Insulin glargine	peakless long-lasting insulin
70/30	premixed solution of fast- and long-acting insulin

Conventional dosing. The most common way of dosing is combining a fast-acting and long-acting insulin several times daily to provide 24 hours of coverage. The graph below shows how regular insulin (short acting) and NPH insulin (long acting) would cover a 24-hour day.

Breakfast   Lunch   Dinner   Bedtime

R   R

N   N

The regular and NPH insulin taken at breakfast are in charge of the glucose numbers at lunch and at dinner. The regular insulin taken at dinner is in charge of the bedtime number. And the NPH insulin taken at bedtime controls the waking or breakfast blood sugar the following morning. Saying that the insulin is in charge of the glucose means that we are hoping that insulin will bring your glucose back in range before you eat your next meal. It will not cover that meal, just have you in range before eating it.

Conventional dosing requires you to have consistent amounts of food (especially carbohydrate) at mealtimes, not skip meals, and stay on a fairly regular time schedule. Conventional dosing is used most commonly in children and adults who have a fairly set schedule. It does not work well for people with multiple work or school schedules, or for people who are very inconsistent with meal timing and food intake. Premixed vials of R and NPH or of Humalog or Novolog (fast-acting insulins) and NPH can be prescribed for easier dosing.

Multiple daily injections (MDI). MDI dosing requires multiple injections (four or more) of a fast-acting insulin to cover food intake and the use of a very long-acting insulin to cover other insulin needs, such as for sugar put out by the liver and different hormones. You will see insulins called Humalog or Novolog (rapid) combined with injections of an insulin called Ultralente (long-lasting). The graph below shows how Humalog and Ultralente would cover a 24-hour day.

Breakfast   Lunch   Dinner   Bedtime

H   H   H   H

U   U

With MDI dosing, Ultralente insulin is given as a basal, or background, insulin. It does not cover food as the other insulins do; rather, it is a very low-profile insulin that provides only the basic metabolic insulin needs—insulin to cover the sugar released from the liver or from other hormones. When you do eat, you must take a shot of fast-acting insulin every time. That means that if you have eight meals a day, you must take eight different shots of Humalog or Novolog. Rapid-acting insulin works very fast to cover the meal, but it does not last long enough to cover two meals.

Why would someone choose eight or more shots compared to two? Flexibility. With MDI you can pretty much eat whatever you want, whenever you want, as long as you count the amount of carbohydrates (carbs) you are eating and take the appropriate amount of insulin to cover the carbs. With MDI it is easier to skip or delay a meal, and as long as you have not taken a shot of rapid-acting insulin, you are not committed to eating anything.

On the flip side, this would not be a good choice for some children who are afraid of injections, or those who would stop eating just to avoid a shot. It is also not a good option if you have difficulty with basic meal planning, carb counting, or drawing up and giving your own insulin. It allows for more flexibility, but it also requires more discipline and responsibility. With MDI, you must always have insulin with you in some form, and you need to monitor blood sugar levels before eating anything. Keep in mind that if you eat everything you want, you will gain weight rapidly. Good nutrition is always a priority.

Again, there are many different ways to use insulin. With the conventional method you can take extra rapid-acting insulin to allow for extra food at special occasions. It can also be used anytime to bring down a high blood sugar. NPH insulin is often used at night in combination with diabetes pills to correct the "dawn phenomenon," an automatic rise in early morning glucose. Whichever method you use, the goal is to have your blood sugars within range most of the time, across the day.

QUESTIONS

*Why can't I take enough medication or insulin to control my
blood sugar and forget about following a meal plan?*

Once again, diabetes is not that simple. First of all, good
nutrition and meal planning are important for everyone, not just
people with diabetes. Second, the medication you take will work
better with meal planning, and will be less effective without meal
planning. And third, you can out-eat any medication, no matter how
fabulous it is. Your medications are adjusted according to your usual
or recommended meal plan. If you eat differently every day, it will
be very difficult to adjust your medications, your glucose levels will
fluctuate more, and you will exhaust the insulin-producing cells you
do have. In the long run you will require more and more medication
to obtain the same glucose results. Following a daily meal plan most
of the time is the number one thing you can do to help your medications work better and to manage your diabetes in the best way
you can.

If food is so essential, why am I on a diet?

Since every cell in the body needs 24-hour-a-day nutrition and a body with diabetes struggles to use food properly, ensuring that you get the most out of what you eat is essential. Remember, everything you eat will be broken down for sugar for the cells. Following a meal plan has many benefits in addition to feeding the cells, however. It provides a tool for weight management and cholesterol management, assures adequate nutrition for wound healing and growth, enhances the effect of medications, helps restore glucose storage in the body, and provides enjoyment. But everything you eat will also raise the blood sugar level differently, so it is important to know the basic food groups and their effects on blood glucose, and to have a meal plan calculated to balance them all.

Meal Plans

A meal plan needs to be specific to you—*one size does not fit all.* Preplanned calorie diets lead to boredom, frustration, and a loss of flexibility. They are mostly ineffective and are usually abandoned soon after starting. A meal plan needs to be built on your needs, likes, and lifestyle; it needs to reflect your ideas and what you are willing to do. If a meal plan does this, you are more likely to stick with it and have success. A dietitian can estimate your calorie and carbohydrate needs and formulate them into a meal plan that works for you.

Carbohydrates, Proteins and Fats

All the food you eat can be broken down into three main nutrients: carbohydrates, proteins, and fats. Carbohydrates have the greatest and most immediate effect on the blood sugar and are the first source of energy for the body. Protein is needed for growth and tissue maintenance and is the second energy source for the body. Protein has a delayed and prolonged effect on the blood sugar. Fats function as slow or stored energy sources. They have little immediate effect on blood sugar levels and are high in calories. When I was diagnosed with diabetes 27 years ago, we did not understand the relationship between carbohydrate and blood sugar levels. I was taught to avoid foods that had added or refined sugar because we thought that was what raised the blood sugar level. We did not understand that every carbohydrate turns into sugar in the body.

With our present knowledge about carbohydrates, we have more flexibility in meal planning than ever before. Moreover, we can eliminate the terms "cheating" and "sneaking" from our meal-planning vocabulary. A dietitian can estimate the amount of carbo-hydrate (carb) you need per meal or snack, and you can choose where those carbs come from. Try not to become so focused on carb counting that you forget good general nutrition; all food groups are important. The carbohydrates simply affect your blood sugar more, so keeping them consistent will make a big difference in glucose pattern management. The following list gives you a general idea of which foods contain carbohydrate. Portion sizes are found on labels, in nutritional count books, and in the American Diabetes Association and the American Dietetic Association's *Exchange Lists for Meal Planning* (Table 7-1).

TABLE 7-1. CARB COUNTING BASICS

Bread/starches/pasta per serving *(1 slice or 1/2 cup)*	=	15 g carb
Fruits per serving *(Specific to fruit or juice)*	=	15 g carb
Milk per 1 cup serving	=	12 g carb
Starchy vegetables per serving *(1/2 cup cooked)*	=	15 g carb
Cooked vegetables per serving *(1/2 cup cooked)*	=	5 g carb
Raw vegetables per serving *(1 cup raw)*	=	5 g carb
Meats/protein per 1 oz serving	=	0 carb
Fats per serving	=	0 carb
Free foods per one serving	=	<5 g carb

A free food is any food with fewer than 20 calories or 5 grams of carb per serving. Typically, one or two free choices a day, not consumed at the same time, will have minimal effect on a blood sugar level.

With Exchange information and the information you can get off food labels, you will find foods that have the same amount of carbohydrate, so you can substitute them into your meal plan to give you more variety. For example, all the following foods have the same amount of carbohydrate:

1/2 cup juice = 1 slice of bread = 2 Oreo cookies = 4 Starburst's candies = 1/2 cup of corn = 3 cups plain popcorn = 1 cup milk = 20 Teddy Grahams

All these choices have the same amount of carbohydrate, so they will affect the blood sugar similarly, but they do not have equal nutritional value. Your body may not know if your sugar level is rising because of a candy bar or a glass of juice, but that's not the whole picture. You eat food for fuel and to get the vitamins and minerals in the food so your body will run well and be healthy. Some highly processed foods don't have any vitamins and minerals to give you. Their calories are "empty" calories.

If you have a hard time following a meal plan. Ask yourself: Do I understand it? Does it fit my lifestyle? Am I trying to change too many things at once? If you answered "yes" to any of these questions, work closely with your dietitian to change just one or two things at a time. Set simple, specific goals. Do not try to give up all foods with sugar or fat in them. Instead, pick one eating habit to change at a time. For example, rather than giving up your favorite cold cereal, start by only having one bowl instead of two or three. Choose one food item that you know you eat too much of, such as cashews, mini-cookies, or mints, and stop buying that item. Every little change makes a difference. And as you succeed more often, you build your confidence to make other changes. Give everything an honest try. For example, before you refuse to try fat-free butter, try a couple of different brands. Some are better than others. Or try mixing a cup of butter with a cup of canola oil to make your own butter spread and avoid the trans fats in hydrogenated oils (found in margarine and store-bought foods such as cookies or crackers).

Food records. Your dietitian may ask you to keep a food record for several days. Writing down what you eat is a real eye-opener. You can identify your actual eating habits, see how serving sizes grow, and how all the little snacks add up. It is the little things that lead to weight gain and poor glucose management.

Healthy and Helpful Snacking Ideas

* Make fruits and vegetables more visible and treats *less* visible, because what you see is often what you eat. If candy bars are sitting in front of you, you will want them; if baby carrots are sitting in front of you, you will eat them.

- Taste your food before you salt it, add additional spices before salt, and use salt substitutes. These will all help to keep blood pressure down if you are sensitive to salt.

- Dip your fork in dressing rather than pouring the dressing on your salad. This will decrease the amount you use and help you cut back on fat. Do the same with syrup.

- I find that when I dip graham crackers in milk, I can eat an entire package without even thinking about it. That is because the milk softens the cracker so much I do not have to chew anything. If you like crackers and milk, take out the serving of crackers and put away the rest so you will not keep eating.

- Crackers dipped in low-fat cottage cheese or peanut butter take longer to eat and are more filling than crackers dipped in milk.

- Do not snack in front of the TV or in your car. It is amazing the number of calories you can take in when you are concentrating on something other than what you are chewing.

- Have a glass or two of water before or with each snack; it helps you feel fuller.

- Use smaller plates, **eat slowly**, put your fork down between bites, and drink water before each meal.

- Do not socialize by the food table. It is too tempting to keep eating as you visit.

- Don't skip meals, it doesn't help you lose weight. Skipping meals slows down your metabolism. Eating on a regular schedule keeps your energy level higher and your metabolism going, and helps your body use calories more effectively.

- Eat slowly. When you eat too fast, you usually eat too much before you feel full.

- When you go to a convenience store to get a soda pop, use the drive-up window if there is one; then you will not see all the goodies inside and decide to buy those also.

Here are some additional tricks of the trade I have discovered for solving meal planning issues.

Breakfast Help

- Premeasure cereal into plastic resealable bags. This keeps your portions from growing and saves time measuring in the morning.

- If you like a lot of cereal, try to eat more of the puffier cereals, such as puffed wheat or puffed rice. You can usually have two to three times as much as you can flaked or sugar-coated cereals. Add some Nutra-Sweet to your puffed wheat, and it will taste like Super Sugar Crisp!

- Use reduced-fat Bisquick and eggs or some kind of egg replacer to make pancakes, waffles, or biscuits. You can freeze them and take out only the amount you need when it's mealtime.

- An excellent sugar-free syrup is Cary's sugar-free syrup—it's my favorite!

Egg replacers. Egg Beaters can be used in any recipe that calls for eggs. You can also use them for scrambled eggs or omelets. By using Eggs Beaters instead of eggs, you'll add no fat or cholesterol, if that is a concern for you.

Butter. Try using the nonstick sprays and low-fat or no-fat butters.

Spreads. If you use the light, low-fat, and or fat-free mayonnaise; sour cream; cream cheese; or salad dressings, you can usually have two to three times as much. But do keep in mind that if you are eating two to three times as much, you really aren't saving any calories. Check the carb count of low-fat products. It is usually higher than in the regular version of the food.

Juices. If you like to drink lots of juice, make up a gallon of Crystal Light and add to that a six-ounce can of frozen orange juice, properly diluted in water. You can have three cups of this compared to one-half cup of regular juice—and it tastes great. You can also buy Twister Light and Ocean Spray Light juice drinks.

Gravy. If you use the packaged gravy mixes from the store, you can have as much as you want, because most of them are fat-free and carb-free. Be aware, however, that they are high in salt. An easy way to skim fat from meat drippings is to pour the juices into a plastic resealable bag. The juices will go to the bottom and the fat will rise to the top. Holding the bag over a pan or bowl, cut one of the bottom corners off and let the juices run out. It works great! Add the juices to the packaged mixes for even better flavor.

Meats. Instead of frying meat or using creamed soups, try Shake'n Bake or Oven Fry coating for chicken and pork; they add no fat and taste good. You can have a thicker, crunchier flavor if you first dip your meat in Egg Beaters.

Casseroles. Use Healthy Choice low-fat plain or creamed soups and light or fat-free sour cream to decrease the fat content. Check the carb count of each product you use.

Mashed potatoes. Flavor with chicken broth or Butter Buds instead of butter, and it is fat free!

Chocolate milk. No Sugar Added Nesquik (formerly Nestlé Quik), is great for a nighttime snack, because mixed with milk it provides both carbohydrate and protein. It can also be added to Cool Whip Lite to make chocolate frosting.

Popcorn. You can have a lot of popcorn (3 cups) for a low amount of carbohydrate, but it can be very high in fat. Use the light microwave popcorn, or butter your popcorn with "I Can't Believe It's Not Butter" spray. You can also make flavored popcorn by sprinkling on dry sugar-free Kool Aid or Jell-O over warm popcorn.

Chips. Use the baked chips instead of fried varieties. There are also WOW brand tortilla chips, and ripple and regular chips that are fat-free.

Dips. When dipping chips or vegetables, salsa is a free food choice. Other dips can be extremely high in fat. If you are making your own vegetable dip, use the low-fat or fat-free sour cream or cream cheeses. For fruit dips use fat-free, sugar-free yogurt. It is low in carbohydrate and a great protein source.

Desserts. Any recipe that calls for Cool Whip, Jell-O, or pudding can be made sugar-free and often fat-free by using the sugar-free Jell-O pudding or Cool Whip Lite.

Candy. If you eat a lot of sugar-free candies, you may have horrible diarrhea and stomach cramps. Plus, they often turn into sugar in the body. Many of the sugar-free candies are made with Sorbitol, a natural laxative. Foods sweetened with Nutra-Sweet or Aspartame usually do not have these side effects. Breath Savers and Velamints are excellent hard candies that do not seem to cause stomach upset.

Cool Whip Lite. Cool Whip Lite can be used for just about everything. When it is frozen, it tastes just like vanilla ice cream, but it is a free food. Have a Diet Coke or rootbeer float using Cool Whip Lite; both are completely free. You can also put a scoop of frozen Cool Whip in sugar-free hot chocolate to sweeten it up a bit. Cool Whip sugar-free yogurt, and lite cream cheese make a great fruit salad dressing or fruit dip. Frosting can be made with Cool Whip Lite and sugar-free pudding mixes, Jell-O, or No Sugar Added Nesquik. You can top all desserts with Cool Whip Lite, and frost cakes, cookies, or graham crackers with it.

Food Cravings

My best advice is: Give in once in a while. Occasionally have what you enjoy; otherwise you will feel angry and controlled by your diabetes. Take control of the situation ahead of time, however: decide what you want to eat, how much is safe, and what other changes you can make in your meal plan to accommodate what you crave. For example, pass up two rolls at dinner if you want dessert. Do not tell yourself you cannot have a favorite treat. Such restriction gives diabetes too much power. Instead, tell yourself something like "I choose not to have chocolate fudge because I want to have more of something else," or "I'm going to enjoy this piece of fudge, and afterwards I'm going to enjoy a walk." By using this self-talk, you can still enjoy your favorite treats from time to time.

Patients ask me all the time, "I'm starving. Isn't there anything I can just eat without worrying?" I have found a few solutions that work for me, aside from the good old diet drinks.

Popcorn Jell-O. Make up three or four different kinds of sugar-free Jell-O in different bread tins. When the Jell-O is well set, cut it into tiny cubes, then mix them all together. Eat them one at a time, just like popcorn shrimp or chicken. No carbohydrates and no calories! It sounds crazy, but it works. I have found that if I do not add all the water the Jell-O calls for, the cubes hold their shape better.

Diet Coke float. I have mentioned this one before, but it is one of my favorites. Add a scoop of frozen Cool Whip Lite to Diet Coke or diet rootbeer. It tastes just like an ice cream float, but it's a free choice! Make sure it is not the regular Cool Whip, which is made with refined sugar and saturated fat.

Fluffy Jell-O. This recipe has a dozen different names. Combine one large container of low-fat cottage cheese with one package of dry, sugar-free Jell-O and 8 ounces of Cool Whip Lite. Mix together well and chill. The cottage cheese counts as protein, which has little effect on the blood sugar, while the Cool Whip Lite and Jell-O are free choices. You can also add fruit, but then you need to count the carbohydrate in the fruit. It still goes a long way!

Shopping Tricks

- Go food shopping after you have eaten, not on an empty stomach. If you are hungry when you shop, it is hard not to give in to your appetite.

- If you are craving something sweet, get a 25-cent gumball to chew on while you shop. It might be hard to talk, but it cures a sweet craving and only has about 5 grams of carbohydrate.

- Buy treats in single-serve packages rather than in large packages. The more treats you have accessible to you, the more you will be tempted to eat. And even though they may be bite-size pieces, they all add up after you eat five or six or seven.

- I like to pretend my patients are all watching me shop, so I try to set a good example. Set a good example for someone. Sure enough, if you buy a lot of things you probably should not have, the "diabetes police" will be there.

- Do not buy chocolates, candies, or cookies for your kids or grandchildren. They get enough already, and you will end up eating them too. Chop up fruit or vegetables and have them sitting out instead. They're better for all of you.

- Do not spend extra money buying sugar-free ice cream or cookies. These items usually have the same amount of carbohydrate, or more, and they cost a lot more.

- Be a label reader. Take notice. If a label says the product is fat-free, it is usually higher in carbohydrate or sugar. If the label says the product is sugar-free or low-sugar, it may still have tons of carbohydrate, which all turns into sugar in the body. Often you will find that low-sugar foods are also higher in fat.

QUESTIONS

I have heard that the diabetes meal plan and diabetes medications will make me gain weight. Is this true?

When your blood sugars are high, your kidneys filter out sugar (calories), and this may keep you from gaining weight or even help you lose weight. But when you start on a meal plan and take diabetic medications, your blood sugar is in range, and you stop losing calories in the urine. There may be some weight gain. This is another reason to add exercise to your diabetes care plan—to use up those calories. Improved glucose control, with or without medication, is the only way we know to prevent complications. So if you are gaining weight with better control, review your meal plan with your dietitian, increase your physical activity, find ways to cope with stress other than eating, and believe that you will succeed.

Since we are talking about weight, consider this weight-loss perspective. Quick weight loss always sounds better than slow weight loss. But research shows that weight taken off slowly and consistently is more likely to stay off. I like to think of it this way: It takes 3,500 calories to lose one pound. By cutting back only 500 calories a day, you will lose one pound a week. That works out to be 52 pounds a year. I can do that! But remember, you can easily eat those calories back in one big meal.

I have heard that protein is hard on the kidneys and should be avoided. Is this true?

Avoiding protein is not necessary unless you have diagnosed kidney disease. And contrary to what many diet books say, protein does require some insulin to be utilized by the body. Protein may be lower in carbohydrate, so it has less of an effect on the blood sugar, but on the other hand, many proteins are high in fat, which contributes to increased weight, cholesterol, and blood fat levels. These factors all lead to decreased insulin effectiveness. There is a great deal of controversy over protein diets. Consult your dietitian for accurate information. Recommended daily intake of protein is 0.8g/kg body weight, or 10 to 20% of daily calories.

What is the difference between sugar alcohols and noncaloric sugar substitutes?

Sugar alcohols are sweeteners that are used instead of sugar. They have two or three calories per gram, whereas sugar has four calories per gram. They are absorbed more slowly and may have less effect on blood sugars than real sugar, but they can also cause gastrointestinal problems. Noncaloric sugar substitutes are sweeteners that do not raise blood sugar levels. NutraSweet, Equal, Sugar Twin, Splenda, Sweet 1, and Sweet 'N Low all are non-caloric sweeteners that are some of my favorites. Honey, fructose, corn syrup, or fruit juices all have carbohydrate and must be counted in your meal planning.

My cholesterol level is high too. What can I do about that?

Your liver makes most of the cholesterol in your body, but foods that are high in cholesterol also contribute to it. If your cholesterol or blood fat levels are high, increase your physical activity, which will help you lose weight, and avoid high saturated-fat foods. Choose soft tub butters or spreads instead of stick butters, sprays instead of oil, and baked products instead of fried. Eating more high-fiber foods and vegetables can also help.

Chapter 8

I thought diabetes meant high blood sugar. Why should I worry about blood sugars going too low?

When you were diagnosed with diabetes, you inherited the job of blood sugar control. But no matter how perfect you are in meal planning, exercise, or medications, you still cannot be as good as your pancreas used to be. You may over- or under-medicate, overeat or under-eat, or exercise more than usual. Remember also that many hormones in your body affect blood sugar levels, and you do not have any control over that. Because of all these factors, you may experience blood sugar levels that go too high or too low. Be prepared to recognize and treat both. Hypoglycemia or low blood sugars can occur when glucose levels drop below 70 mg/dl.

SYMPTOMS OF HYPOGLYCEMIA

The symptoms of mild hypoglycemia come on quickly and can be compared to the feelings you experience when waking up from a nightmare. Shaking, sweating, pounding heart, anxiety, crying, panic, and vision distortions are all common symptoms. You may have symptoms that are unique just to you. I will start to yawn over and over, or I will get tingling sensations in my face and thighs. Sometimes my arms will feel like they weigh 2,000 pounds each. These symptoms come on over several minutes. Chances are that if you can sense a change coming over you, it may be hypoglycemia. Moderate to severe hypoglycemia symptoms may include confusion, staggering, lethargy, unconsciousness, and seizures. The longer a person has diabetes, the tighter controlled their blood sugars are, and the older they are, the fewer symptoms they may have to alert them of hypoglycemia. This is why it is critical to always have something with you to treat hypoglycemia as soon as you, or someone else, recognize the symptoms.

The 15/15 treatment rule. When you make punch and it is not sweet enough, you add sugar. You need to do the same thing for a low blood sugar—add sugar. Treatment of a low blood sugar involves eating about 10–15 grams of carbohydrate (see below). After about 15 minutes, you can recheck the glucose level to see if it has come up enough.

Usually you can tell by how you are feeling whether the treatment is working or not. Some carbohydrate foods are better than others for treating lows. You do not have to buy something special just to treat hypoglycemia, but convenience does help. The carbohydrate you use to treat a low blood sugar does not have to be subtracted from your next meal. It is independent. However, if you are low at a meal time, just eat your meal, and you will get enough carbohydrate to bring your sugar level up.

Easy-treatment carbohydrates. Many foods have carbohydrate or sugar in them. You could eat an orange, chew regular gum, or have a sandwich. But sometimes your blood sugar is low enough that you do not have the strength or time to peel and section an orange or chew a sandwich. In these times, you need something simple, convenient, and quick. A better choice might be 4 ounces of juice, three glucose tablets, a glass of milk, or 6 ounces of regular soda pop. There is also less risk of choking when you use liquids.

In a pinch, you could use many things in your kitchen, such as frozen juice concentrate, table sugar, syrup, brown sugar, powdered sugar, honey, jam, jelly, or cake frosting. All these items will raise the blood sugar quickly. Special products are made for treating hypoglycemia that are a little more convenient to carry with you, such as glucose tablets or gel. They can be found at any pharmacy and purchased without a prescription. It takes three to four glucose tablets to equal 15 grams of carbohydrate. Read the label on the product.

If a blood sugar becomes low enough, you may not be able to talk, walk, or communicate; you may be confused or want to fight. In this situation it is not safe to use food that requires chewing and coordination in swallowing. A safer choice in this case would be the glucose gels. These can be squeezed into the cheek or inside the lip and even if not swallowed, some of it will be absorbed through the gums and the tongue. Then when you are more alert, you can be treated with something more substantial. Untreated hypoglycemia can lead to seizures and loss of consciousness. In this situation nothing should be put in your mouth. Glucagon should be injected or 911 called.

The problem with chocolate and candy. When I was diagnosed with diabetes 27 years ago, I was taught to eat a candy bar if I felt low. Now that we know more about nutrition and how fast different foods digest, we know that foods high in fat often digest slower than those with just carbohydrate or sugar, such as a glass of fruit juice or nonfat milk. When your blood sugars are low, you need something that will raise the blood sugar quickly. Many times when we eat a candy bar, we still do not feel better after several minutes, so we eat or drink something else. Then when everything has had time to digest, we find ourselves with the opposite problem, high blood sugar.

The problem with candy is not that it is too high in fat; it is just too hard to stop eating it. I know exactly how many Skittles or Starbursts I need to get 15 grams of carbohydrate. But when my blood sugar is low, 12 Skittles are not going to cut it. I want the whole bag. I also know that if I have some kind of candy in my car to treat lows, I will likely feel low whether I am or not, just so I can have some of that candy. If you have will power and can stop after 15 grams, candy is an acceptable treatment.

Same blood sugar level—different symptoms. A patient once told me he had a blood sugar of 50 one day and had no symptoms at all. The next day, however, he woke up when his wife was squirting glucose gel into his mouth. His blood sugar at that time was 53. He wondered how he could have almost the same blood sugar level and yet totally different responses. This is not uncommon. I try to figure out the reason for feeling so different by asking how fast I dropped and how far I have come down. Usually the faster a blood sugar is dropping, the sooner you feel symptoms, and the farther it drops, the more obvious the symptoms are. Consider the following examples.

EXAMPLE 1

Blood sugar at breakfast was 100. By noon it was 60.
(A body can easily compensate for a 40-point drop over four hours; symptoms are mild.)

Blood sugar at breakfast was 300. By noon it was 60.
(This time the blood sugar has dropped 240 points in several hours; the body is more likely to feel this one.)

EXAMPLE 2

Blood sugar at 8:00 a.m. was 100. By noon it was 60.
(Again, a 40-point drop over several hours is no big deal; symptoms are mild.)

Blood sugar at 8:00 a.m. was 100. By 8:20 it was 60.
(The blood sugar now dropped 40 points in only 20 minutes; this may cause significant symptoms.)

Is it common for blood sugars to change so drastically? I would probably be safe in saying "no," if you are not taking insulin injections. But diabetes sticks to few rules, and you are always better off being prepared.

Recommendations for Preventing Lows

Always have something with you to treat hypoglycemia. It seems to work like Murphy's Law: If you don't have something with you to treat a low blood sugar, you can count on going low. If you do have something with you, you will not go low; or if you do, you will be able to treat the problem quickly.

Keep something in your car. If you get stuck in rush-hour traffic, or have a minor car accident, or the freeway gets closed, if your medication is kicking in and it's mealtime, you could have a real problem if you do not have something with you for fuel. I grew up with crackers and juice in the glove compartment of our car. I do the same thing today. I know that if I need something, or if someone else does, I have it with me. My favorite thing to keep in the car is CapriSun fruit juice. It has a little more carbohydrate than I need, but it can be in my car year round and not go bad. Hot or cold, it stores well and works great.

If in doubt, treat. Sometimes the symptoms of high and low blood sugar may feel the same to you. If you are unsure about your symptoms and you have no meter to check with, the safest thing is to treat for a low blood sugar. If you are low, you have just treated the problem and in a few minutes you will begin to feel better. If you are low and decide to wait until you get home to check your blood sugar, you may not make it home before having severe hypoglycemia. If you are high and you go ahead and treat for a low, the worst thing that is going to happen is that your blood sugar will go a little bit higher than it already is, and this is not an emergency. High blood sugars can be treated when you get home.

Check your blood sugar ASAP. Some of the symptoms of high and low blood sugars may feel the same, so you are always better off monitoring than guessing. If low blood sugars are a frequent problem at a certain time of day, you may need a medication change. Sometimes you will find that your blood sugars are not really low; your symptoms may be the result of hunger, anxiety, or stress, or a rapid swing in blood sugar.

Have a snack if a meal will be late or missed. Sometimes situations come up when your medication is kicking in or you have taken it, and then you cannot eat. Do the same thing you would do for a young child. Eat a snack that will tide you over. For example, if you forgot to turn the oven on and dinner won't be ready for several hours, have a snack that includes some carbohydrate as well as protein. Have a breakfast drink, a glass of milk, or half a sandwich, something more substantial than 4 ounces of juice.

Hypoglycemia Unawareness

Hypoglycemia unawareness refers to those times when you have no symptoms to alert you to a low blood sugar. It is more common among people who have had diabetes for many years and among those who keep their blood sugars low and have frequent hypoglycemic episodes. Hypoglycemia unawareness can also be the result of autonomic neuropathy (nerve damage to the body's automatic processes) or beta blocker use. Both autonomic neuropathy and beta blockers can decrease the warning signs of hypoglycemia, as well as decrease the liver's release of glucose. Checking blood sugars more frequently and making an effort to avoid even mild hypoglycemia will help keep hypoglycemia unawareness from worsening.

QUESTIONS

What if I feel low, but I check my blood sugar and I am not low?

Several things can be happening that may mimic the symptoms of hypoglycemia.

What does your body think a normal blood sugar is? If your body is used to running in the 300s because you did not know you had diabetes, then when you bring it down into a normal range, you may feel low. It takes some time, but you need to retrain your body so that a normal blood sugar feels better than a high blood sugar.

Are you dropping? Sometimes I check my blood sugar, and it says 85, not low enough to cause symptoms for me. So if I really feel as if something is going on, I will recheck my blood sugar in 5 to 10 minutes. If it has dropped 10 to 15 points, I know I am on the way down. I think everyone with diabetes becomes familiar with this sensation or the expression "I'm dropping."

Have you gone a long time without eating? If you have gone for an extended time without eating, even if your blood sugars are not significantly low, your body needs fuel. Symptoms such as shakiness, headache, or extreme fatigue are ways the body sends a message to you to feed it.

Could your symptoms not be related to diabetes? Stress, anxiety, tension, and even certain over-the-counter medications, such as decongestants, may make you feel as if you are low. Withdrawal from medications, mild allergic reactions, fear, and certain stimulants can also feel like hypoglycemia.

What happens if I have a low blood sugar while I'm asleep?

Usually a low blood sugar during the night will wake you up. It may take a minute to figure out why you are awake, but you will tune into the fact that your heart is pounding, or you are sweating and shaking. Symptoms that would alert you to lows during the night might also include waking up with a headache, falling out of bed, having nightmares, restless sleep, or waking up exhausted.

What happens if a low blood sugar goes untreated?

Many people think that a low blood sugar untreated will result in death. This outcome is extremely rare. The body has many ways of protecting itself from low blood sugars. Once again, your hormones kick in. When your blood sugars go low for an extended period, your body releases stress hormones, such as glucagon and epinephrine (adrenaline). These stress hormones all naturally raise the blood sugar. Glucagon from the pancreas tells the liver to release stored sugar. The hormone epinephrine tells the liver to convert stored nutrients into more glucose. Sometimes the body will go into seizures, making the muscles take up more glucose and making the hypoglycemia worse.

Chapter 9

Exercise: your "rite" to good health

Exercise can be one of the toughest things to do consistently, next to eating correctly, but it is just as important. Exercise can be used instead of medication to lower blood sugar, and it improves your body's response to the medications you do take by unlocking the "deadbolts" on your cell doors. Exercise improves every aspect of your physical and mental health, and best of all, it is free. Your body needs regular exercise to function properly. A colleague of mine tells his patients that the body is the only machine that breaks down when we do not use it. That is so true—we need to use it or lose it.

Usually, the more physically active you are, the less medication you have to take for all kinds of problems. Look at all the illnesses we take medication for that could be helped with exercise.

Exercise Can Mean Less Medications

- Exercise relieves stress and anxiety—decreasing the need for tranquilizers and anti-anxiety medications.

- Exercise lowers blood pressure—decreasing the need for blood pressure medications.

- Exercise lowers blood sugars—decreasing the need for insulin or pills to treat diabetes.

- Exercise helps you sleep better—no need for sleeping pills.

- Exercise increases energy during the day—without the side effects of stimulants.

- Exercise improves self-esteem and decreases depression—decreasing the need for antidepressant medications.

- Exercise decreases muscle aches and stiffness—so you don't use anti-inflammatory drugs, muscle relaxants, or painkillers.

- Exercise helps you lose weight—so you don't need weight-loss drugs.

- Exercise improves body shape and builds muscles—so you don't need protein drinks to increase muscles.

- Exercise decreases appetite—no need for appetite suppressants.

- Exercise lowers cholesterol—decreasing the need for cholesterol-lowering medications.

- Exercise improves circulation—decreasing the need for circulatory medications.

- Exercise increases bone density and strength—decreasing the loss of calcium from bones.

- Exercise improves your complexion—no need for acne medications and agents to clean pores.

I still have to convince myself occasionally that exercise *can* be one of the fun things I do; it is all in how I look at it. It is easy to come up with reasons not to exercise, and I have come up with them all. As easy as it is to talk myself out of exercising, it is not that easy to build my esteem after I have given in to making excuses. When I finish some physical activity, I feel great. I know I have helped my body and improved my health. Sometimes I even like it when someone sees me walking and later congratulates me for being healthy. It does not work for me to exercise because I am supposed to, or just because I have diabetes. I had to search within me to find reasons to exercise that fulfilled a need of mine.

Exercise is a healthy addiction. I found that when I walked, I saw people and waved to them, and that lifted my spirit. When I walked, I could talk out my frustrations from a hard day at work. My mind became clearer and problems that seemed out of my control suddenly had solutions. I have also found that when I walk, I do not dwell on discouraging or depressing matters. Exercise elevates my mood and improves my outlook on life. It also makes a huge difference if I have someone to walk or exercise with.

Find a reason to exercise that works *for you*, rather than exercising just because you are supposed to. See if any of the following benefits ring true for you.

General Health Benefits of Exercise

- Exercise decreases blood pressure.

- Exercise increases circulation.

- Exercise improves the functions of muscles, bones, ligaments, and tendons.

- Exercise increases your resistance to illness.

- Exercise increases the oxygen to muscles, which serves as fuel for them.

- Exercise increases flexibility and improves posture and appearance.

- Exercise increases blood supply to muscles and organs.

- Exercise decreases the risk of back injury.

- Exercise burns body fat and builds muscle.

Health Benefits of Exercise for People with Diabetes

- Exercise lowers blood sugar levels.

- Exercise reduces the risk of heart disease.

- Exercise improves metabolism.

- Exercise improves glucose tolerance.

- Exercise helps with appetite control.

- Exercise stimulates circulation to narrowed blood vessels.
- Exercise improves insulin sensitivity.
- Exercise decreases elevated blood fat levels.
- Exercise increases the number of cell "doors" for glucose to get in.
- Exercise decreases the risk of complications from diabetes.
- Exercise decreases the amount of medication you need to control your blood glucose.
- Exercise counteracts the effects of obesity.
- Exercise prevents or delays the onset of type 2 diabetes.

Real-Life Benefits of Exercise

- Exercise makes you feel good!
- Exercise is doing something just for you.
- Exercise lengthens your life expectancy.
- Exercise improves your mental alertness and memory.
- Exercise improves your complexion.
- Exercise decreases wrinkles (well, it might!).
- Exercise improves your sense of well-being.
- Exercise improves depression.
- Exercise allows you to work harder and longer with less fatigue.
- Exercise gets you out of the "same old routine."

When you have found a reason or several reasons to exercise, here are a few extra tips to keep you going.

Exercise Tips

Start slowly and work your way up. If you push yourself too hard the first few days, your body will ache and you will not want to continue. If you want to push without hurting yourself, start by doing several short activities several times a day. Over time, increase the length of the activity until you have succeeded in exercising for the time span you would like. Remember, anything you do is going to improve your well-being.

Set realistic goals. If you have never exercised regularly before, do not overwhelm yourself with unrealistic expectations. Start with short exercise episodes several times a day, or even just one. Set a goal to walk to the end of the driveway or to the mailbox. Then add to that distance. I have one patient who set a goal to start exercising one minute every day. Her reasoning was perfect—if she took the time to start, get dressed, and go outside, she knew she would exercise for at least a minute (so she could have success) and most likely for longer. And she was right. Within two weeks she was exercising 45 to 60 minutes a day, and she looked forward to it.

Have some incentives or rewards. Sometimes weight loss or improved strength takes several weeks to show, so reward yourself more often for the exercise you do each day. Take a longer bath, call a friend, play an extra game of solitaire, have an extra diet drink, or go to a movie. When you can walk far enough or long enough to get to the library, treat yourself to a book or tape to listen to while you walk!

Do something different. Do something silly. Make exercise fun. It does not matter how you look, if it keeps you exercising, *keep doing it.* I would set rules for myself. Every time I walked and a car passed me, I would change my stride or whatever I was doing with my arms. If someone honked and waved at me, I would speed up my pace until the next light pole. If I walked by a library or a public building that had stairs, I would climb the stairs, even if there were only two. Take a basketball and bounce it as you walk, try not to step on any cracks, or try to find difficult addresses. Dance, skip, hop, jump—do it. If you make your routine fun, you are more likely to continue it.

How Should I Exercise and How Much Should I Do?

There are several important parts to exercise: the warm-up and cool-down periods and the actual exercise itself. Before starting to exercise, do at least five minutes of warm-up. Warming up increases blood flow to the muscles, which warms them and prevents them from being injured when you stress them. Warming up includes walking, swinging your arms, and gently loosening all muscles of the body—not hard bouncing or jerking.

Adults are encouraged to do 45 to 60 minutes of aerobic exercise five to six times a week. Even if you have never exercised and no matter how old you are, exercise works to make you fit and healthy. Aerobic exercise includes exercises that are rhythmic and continuous, require oxygen, use large muscles groups, and keep your heart rate up throughout the activity. Examples include walking, swimming, biking, or dancing.

When you begin an aerobic workout, you first burn circulating sugar. After about 15 to 20 minutes, you begin to burn stored fat. Burning fat means you have burned stored calories, decreased insulin resistance, and helped speed up your metabolism.

Anaerobic exercise works differently in that it does not require oxygen or the continuous use of large muscle groups. It also does not have the same benefit for your heart as aerobic exercise. It was explained to me once that the sports we typically "play" are anaerobic because they require short spurts of energy and do not elevate the heart rate consistently. When we play volleyball, tennis, or baseball, we are usually doing anaerobic activity. Anaerobic exercise can increase strength in specific muscles, but it does not necessarily burn fat, strengthen the heart, or keep the heart rate up enough.

Many calculations can be done to determine if you are raising your heart rate enough, but most do not take into account the medications you may be taking that prevent a rapid heart beat. An easy way to know if you are pushing yourself hard enough, or too hard, is to do a "talk test." If, while exercising, you cannot talk because you cannot catch your breath, you are pushing too hard. Slow down. If, on the other hand, you can sing a song, you are not pushing hard enough. Try speeding up. Let your body tell you how you are doing. If at any time you experience chest pain or shortness of breath, stop the activity and see a physician. If the exercise you are doing is making you miserable or is causing pain, find something else to do, or you probably will not stick with it. Another option is to speak with an exercise physiologist or physical therapist to learn about safe exercises for you.

When you have finished exercising, don't stop abruptly. Slow down and cool down. You can cool down by doing the same things you did to warm up, or by slowing down during the last five minutes of the activity you are doing. The idea is not to go running or walking for 45 minutes and then stop suddenly.

Several recommendations are important to consider before exercising or starting an exercise program.

Talk with your physician before you start an exercise program. Make sure that your heart is okay for an aerobic workout. It might be helpful to see where your cholesterol and lipid levels are before you start your program, and then have them redone in several months to see your progress.

Check your blood sugar before and after exercise. This will help determine the effect of exercise on your blood sugar. If you have never done regular exercise before, and you are not sure how it affects your blood sugars, checking will give you a lot of helpful information. Exercise usually lowers blood sugar, but sometimes it will go up temporarily. Consider the following example.

Let us say you checked your blood sugar before walking, and it was 150 mg/dl. After walking for an hour (do not exercise for a full hour unless you have worked up to it) and cooling down, your blood sugar has dropped to 100 mg/dl. With this information, you have a rough estimate that an hour's worth of activity may drop you 50 points. This is good to know because if your blood sugar is in a normal range (70–120) before exercise, you might go too low if you first do not have a snack. I pointed out in a class one day that this is also helpful on days like Thanksgiving. If your blood sugar is high because of overeating, you can bring it down by going for a walk. Or, as a patient pointed out, you could go for a walk and then come back for seconds. His sense of humor has a point. By being more physically active, you will have more flexibility in meal planning. Be cautious, though. Exercising immediately after eating is not recommended. Your heart is working hard, pumping extra blood to help with the digestion process. Do not overwork it by adding exercise at the same time.

Here is another example:

Let us say you walk for an hour. This time you start with a blood sugar of 150 mg/dl, and when you have finished exercising, your blood sugar has gone up to 219 mg/dl. This is not uncommon in adults. Even though exercise is positive stress for the body, it is still a stress. Sometimes exercise will cause a release of stress hormones, and your blood sugar may go up temporarily. I call this an exercise high. It does not usually require any treatment, because as your body adjusts to having regular physical activity, the exercise high will be lower. If you were to check your blood sugar over the following couple of hours, you would see it come down on its own. The benefit of regular exercise outweighs the concern for this temporary rise in glucose. Exercise can lower your blood glucose for the next 24 hours.

Carry a source of sugar with you to treat hypoglycemia. Exercise has the potential to drop blood sugar too low. If you are prepared with some source of sugar, you will avoid unwanted problems.

Wear a medical alert bracelet or necklace. This identification is not to point you out, it is to help you if you are not able to speak for yourself and are in need of medical help. It does not need to be fancy or expensive. It simply needs to say "diabetes," which will prompt the emergency response team to check your blood sugar level.

Exercise with someone. Exercise is more enjoyable when shared. Plus, you will more likely continue your exercise program if there is someone to encourage you along.

Wear shoes that fit and socks to prevent injuries. As important as exercise is for improving the circulation in your feet, it can also be hazardous if poor-fitting shoes or socks cause injuries, such as blisters. Study the foot-care guidelines in the next chapter of this book.

Don't wear new exercise shoes for prolonged exercise. Breaking in your exercise shoes will increase your foot comfort as well as prevent injury to your feet.

Check your feet after each exercise session for hidden injuries. Since you cannot rely on the nerves in your feet to send your brain accurate information about injuries, it is imperative that you visually scan and touch your feet to check for possible injuries.

Exercising at the same time of day is helpful, but not critical, for glucose management. Remember that exercise enhances and works like medication. If you do it at a different time every day, your blood sugars will respond differently each day. You may find that if you exercise at the same time of day, you may be able to decrease the amount of medication you need at that time of day.

If you have retinopathy (eye disease) or high blood pressure, your physician may encourage you to avoid jarring activities, heavy weight lifting, or bending with your head below your waist. Check with your physician to be sure what you should and should not do.

If your blood sugar is above 300, you may want to think twice about doing aerobic exercise. Aerobic exercise makes your heart pump harder and requires more oxygen. You may want to consult with your physician about the amount of aerobic exercise that is safe and healthful for your situation.

Do not exercise on an empty stomach *if* you have taken your insulin or pills for diabetes. Exercise helps to lower the blood sugar, as do your medications. Therefore, the combination of insulin or pills and exercise, without food on board, could cause severe hypoglycemia. If you like to exercise before breakfast, that is great. Go ahead and exercise at that time. To play it safe, though, take your medications after you have finished your exercise program and when you are ready to eat your meal.

Chapter 10

And what else is there . . . ?

(General health care recommendations)

Foot Care

Think about your feet for a minute. Feet are farthest from the heart, so they receive circulation last. The vessels in the feet are also some of the smallest in the body, so circulation is already challenged. You walk on them your whole life, gravity works against the return of blood from the feet, and then you add elevated blood sugar levels. Over time, this can all lead to decreased circulation to the small vessels and nerves of the feet and toes.

With decreased circulation and high blood sugars, the nerves in the feet become damaged and lose their ability to sense pain, pressure, temperature, or touch correctly. Your feet can become injured more easily, and it very difficult to heal any injuries you do get. The injuries can go unnoticed and untreated until serious complications result.

Poor circulation in your legs may cause (1) cramping when you walk, (2) thin, dry skin, and (3) sores that won't heal. With poor circulation, oxygen and nutrients are not circulated to the injured area to help repair tissue breakdown, and the high blood sugars interfere with the white blood cells' ability to fight off infection.

This complication is the reason diabetes is the leading cause of lower extremity amputations.

If you follow several basic rules of precaution, you can keep your feet well for your lifetime. These rules include the following:

Do not go barefoot. Most foot injuries occur when you are barefoot. Shoes will not prevent all injuries, but certainly, any injury you do get will be less severe if your feet are protected by shoes.

Prevent your feet from becoming dry or cracked. It is a good idea to apply lotion after you bathe or shower, but don't put lotion between your toes or under toenails. Buildup between your toes is what I call my recipe for toe jam. If you combine the lotion between your toes with the lint from your socks, the dirt from your shoe, the heat and sweat from your foot, plus the powder to keep down odor, you have the perfect recipe for toe jam. You also have a perfect breeding ground for fungus and bacteria. After applying lotion to your feet, run a tissue or towel between your toes to get rid of any excess. If you have powder in your shoes for odor control, when you take your shoes off at night, do the same thing. Get rid of anything that does not belong between your toes, no matter how small or insignificant it may seem.

Prevent burns to the feet. Many adults have diabetes a long time before it is diagnosed. This means there may already be some decreased sensation or feeling to your feet. If this is the case, you may not be able to tell if you are being burned. To prevent burns to your feet, avoid soaking your feet in hot water or placing feet on hot water bottles or heating pads. If you need to soak your foot for medical reasons—which still is not recommended—test the water temperature just as you would for a baby: Stick your elbow in first. If you have really cold feet, try wearing an extra pair of socks during the day and a fresh pair of socks while you sleep. When you are watching TV or reading, you can also put a lap blanket on. If you absolutely have to use a heating pad, put it on top of the lap blanket, not on your feet. You want your feet to last a lifetime, so baby them.

Purchase shoes later in the day. Because of gravity, your feet will have more fluid in them later in the day. If you buy shoes in the morning, they may be too small for you the rest of the day. Tight fitting shoes may lead to injury. After you buy new shoes, only wear them for a few hours at a time, and check your feet for red areas or blisters when you take them off.

Check your feet daily. Look for changes in color, blisters, cracked areas, calluses, corns, or any break in the skin that could allow bacteria in. If you cannot see or reach your feet, have someone else look at them for you.

Check your shoes daily. This rule seemed unnecessary to me until several years ago. I still had good sensation in my feet and knew I would be able to feel if there was something wrong in my shoe. Until one morning, as I got ready to go work in my yard, I put my foot into my boot and smashed a mouse. I am not sure who was scared more, me, the mouse, or my cats when I tried to find them and thank them for the present. The idea is not that we want you to be able to feel a nail, tack, or toothpick when you step on it, but that we want to prevent you from having to find it that way. Then it is too late; injury has occurred. Thankfully, my foot was not hurt, but had I checked my boot prior to putting it on, . . . well. If the mouse had bitten me when I checked the boot, my hand would have healed much faster than my foot, and with less risk for infection.

Wear comfortable socks. Avoid wearing tight hose, socks, or garters that might interfere with circulation. Watch out for thick toe seams that can make your shoe too tight or rub a blister. Wear socks that do not make your feet sweat. Sweating can dry out your feet, which leads to cracking of the skin and increased risk for infections. Cotton or combination cotton and acrylic socks absorb moisture better than nylon socks do, and they do not seem to make your feet sweat as much. If you have a pair of socks you just love, but they make you sweat a lot, when you take them off, wash and dry your feet and then apply lotion to prevent cracking.

Use care clipping your toenails. When you cut your toenails, the most important thing to remember is don't cut them so short that you nick or cut the nail bed. By leaving a little bit of nail, you decrease your risk not only of toe injury but also of ingrown toenails. If you cannot see or feel your toes, have someone else trim your nails for you. If you have severe neuropathy and poor circulation, you may need to have a podiatrist do it.

Never perform any kind of surgery on your own foot. If something requires a blade or scalpel, it needs to be done by a doctor. If the doctor nicks you, he can at least get you started on an antibiotic to prevent an infection. If you cut yourself, you often have to wait until there is a problem before something can be done about it. With diabetes, you don't want to wait for the infection to develop. You may have used a razor on your feet for years without any problems; now is a good time to stop before an injury occurs.

Do not smoke tobacco in any form—cigarettes, cigars, or pipes. Smoking shrinks small blood vessels, which adds one more cause for decreased circulation to your feet. Smoking marijuana may also damage your blood vessels.

Do not use any type of acid plaster or liquid on warts. These acid-based chemicals do not distinguish between bad tissue and good tissue. They will break down whatever they touch. Be safe and let a physician treat warts.

Avoid adhesive bandages on your feet. Sometimes adhesives can irritate or pull too harshly on skin and lead to injury. My favorite thing to use on my injured feet is Coban or Vet Wrap. It is similar to an Ace wrap, but it is very thin and will only stick to itself, not you. It is great for holding dressings in place and for wounds in awkward places. Coban can be found at any medical supply store.

Have your physician check your feet. If you want your physician to look at your feet, *and you do*, take your shoes and socks off before the physician comes in the room. If you are sitting there barefooted, the doctor cannot help but see your feet. And just by looking at them, the doctor can tell if your feet are swollen, what color they are, if the nails have problems, or if there are sores or wounds that need attention. Usually, if your shoes and socks are off, this also reminds your physician to feel your feet and check for circulation and sensation with a thin plastic wire called a monofilament.

Be very kind to your feet. Massage them, elevate and rest them, and exercise them. You want them to last your entire life, so cater to their special needs.

Stop foot-care problems before they start. It is easier to treat a foot that does not have infection, poor circulation, or nerve disease. And it is always easier to prevent foot problems than to treat them. If you do receive an injury to your feet, see your physician for the best advice on how to manage it. When he or she says not to walk on the infected foot, don't walk on it. Use crutches, a wheelchair, or bedrest, but staying off the foot is the most important thing you can do for it.

Dental Care

When blood sugar levels are elevated, the mucous membranes of the body are "sugar coated." This means your saliva and mouth have sugar in them. There are many differing opinions on the relationship between dental disease and diabetes, but we do know that when a person with diabetes develops any kind of dental disorder, healing is slower due to the high sugar content of the saliva. This usually has a greater affect on the gums than on the teeth. Poorly controlled diabetes can lead to gum disease, gingivitis, bad breath, slow wound healing, tooth decay, yeast infections, dry mouth, cracked lips, and a decreased sense of taste. Keep in mind that poor oral health is a stress that can lead to higher blood sugars, and higher blood sugars can lead to poor oral health. Good glucose control and proper oral hygiene will help prevent tooth and gum disease.

Dental Do's

- Brush your teeth following meals using a soft, nonabrasive brush.

- Floss between teeth daily.

- Report to your dentist any of the following symptoms: red, irritated, or bleeding gums; frequent or large cankers or ulcers; odor, pain, or swelling; white or yellow patches on gums or tongue.

- Visit your dentist at least every six months and be sure he or she knows you have diabetes.

Eye Care

The longer you have diabetes, the more at risk you are for eye problems. These problems are addressed more in chapter 13, on long-term complications. To catch these problems before they affect your vision, follow these recommendations.

Have a dilated eye exam every year by an eye doctor. This is not a vision check to see whether you need glasses or a change in your prescription; this is to have the blood supply to the back of the eye (retina) checked for damage from the diabetes. This examination is discussed in more detail in chapter 13.

Do not change eyeglass prescriptions when your diabetes is poorly controlled. High blood sugars will cause your vision to change daily. Wait until your blood sugars have been stable for at least a month; otherwise you may get glasses that you do not need.

Tell your eye doctor that you have been diagnosed with diabetes if you already see one for vision care.

Report these to your doctor immediately: sudden changes in vision, loss of vision, blind spots, redness or irritation to the eye or eyelid, or a red or orange tint to your vision.

Skin Care

Your skin has the job of regulating your body temperature and water balance, but it also provides a barrier to bacteria and infection. Breaks in the skin, especially in feet and legs, can be difficult to heal. By taking good care of your skin, you assist it in providing protection to your body.

Skin-Care Guidelines

- Use moisturizing soaps instead of deodorant soaps, which are more drying.

- Apply lotions to skin and feet to prevent cracking, but do not let lotion build up between the toes (see foot care guidelines on p. 77).

- Avoid sunburn, harsh chemicals, and exposure to extremes of heat and cold.

- Do not open blisters or pick at scabs. Keep them clean and covered.

- Wear gloves when doing outdoor work to protect hands.

- Report skin problems, such as rashes, bumps, changes in skin color, boils, or change in the shape, size, or color of a mole.

- Instead of using adhesive bandages that can irritate or tear skin, try Coban (also known as "vet wrap" at Intermountain Farmers Association). Coban has no adhesive and will not stick to the skin, only to itself. It conforms to anything you wrap it around, including very large or very small dressings, and it provides a durable barrier to dirt and pressure.

Vitamins

If your diabetes is well managed, you do not need more vitamins than anyone else. However, many people do not eat well or manage their diabetes well, and so a daily multivitamin is sometimes recommended by a dietitian. You can spend a ton of money on expensive super vitamins and minerals from health stores, but the basic one-a-day vitamins found at your grocery store are fine, too. Mineral deficiencies such as chromium and magnesium are very rare in the United States, and you do not need to replace what you are not short of. An excess of these minerals and vitamins is not better for you, it just makes expensive urine, since your body gets rid of the excess. Work with your dietitian if you have any of the following reasons for which nutritional supplements may be needed: vegetarian or extremely low-calorie dieting, diuretic use, poor calcium intake, or other malabsorption problems.

Travel

There is no reason why a person with diabetes should limit travel plans or cut back on vacationing. Just take a few extra precautions and avoid problems.

- Take extra medication with you in case some is lost or spilled.

- Take a prescription stating that you have diabetes and listing all the medications you use. Each medicine must be in its original packaging with the prescription on it. This saves time and hassles going through customs or security.

- Have identification to help identify you as a person with diabetes, in case of emergency.

- Always have emergency food with you. I tell my patients that the safest person to get stranded with is a person with diabetes, because we always have extra food. The trick is not to munch on high-fat, high-calorie foods throughout your travels. A bag of mini-carrots works great to keep your hands and mouth busy. Extra food can also help compensate for road meals that may not meet your needs.

- When flying, keep your medications and glucose meter with you in your carry-on luggage so there is no chance of things being lost with checked-in luggage.

- If you drive or sit for long periods, your blood sugar levels may elevate. Try doing armchair exercises or pulling over every hour or so to walk for a few minutes. You may want to cut back on calories the day you travel, to compensate for the lack of activity.

- Ask your current physician if he or she knows a physician trained in the care of diabetes in the area you are traveling to.

- If you take insulin and are changing time zones, talk with your physician about switching to multiple injections of a rapid-acting insulin until you get to your destination, then return to your typical routine according to the new time zone.

Alcohol Consumption

Alcohol enhances the action of insulin and also slows the release of sugar from the liver, which can result in hypoglycemia. To avoid possible life-threatening hypoglycemia, eat a meal when you drink, and limit how much you drink. Alcohol is also high in fat, so account for it in your meal plan. Avoid alcohol if you are pregnant, have not eaten, or are taking prescription drugs. No amount of alcohol is safe when you drive.

Recreational Drugs

Having diabetes does not change the facts: **Don't do drugs.** When drugs are involved, diabetes care is disabled or forgotten; medications are missed, and severe hypoglycemia and hyper-glycemia occur. Drugs will complicate any diabetes complications, and diabetes will complicate any drug complication.

Smoking—Just Don't Do It.

Smoking and diabetes is a fatal combination. Smoking decreases the ability of red blood cells to carry oxygen and reduces blood vessel size, which decreases circulation. Smoking increases your risk for every serious complication of diabetes and speeds up the progress of existing complications. Smoking also prevents and slows the healing process when you are sick or injured and has been proven to cause lung and throat cancer.

QUESTIONS

My feet are always cold. What can I do to warm them if I can't use a heating pad?

Several things will help cold feet. First of all, change your socks if they become damp. Socks that are damp, even from sweating, will contribute to cold feet. Dry socks help warm the feet. Try wearing an extra pair of socks during cold weather to provide extra insulation for your feet. When watching TV or reading, place a blanket on your lap so that any blood going to your feet seems warmer. If you can, massage each foot while you're sitting there to increase circulation and warmth in them. You can wear a pair of socks to bed to help with cold feet at night. If your feet are so cold you absolutely have to do something, try sticking a towel in the dryer for a few minutes and then wrap it around your feet. My other suggestion is to exercise your feet when in bed or watching TV. Crinkle up your toes and then stretch them out; do ankle rolls or pretend you are walking—anything that will increase the circulation to your feet will help them feel warmer.

I've heard that you can get horrible foot infections from public swimming pools. Should I avoid swimming because of this?

While it is true—you can get foot infections from public pools—it is good to swim, especially if this is the only form of exercise you can do. The cause of foot fungus or viruses is usually found on the shower or locker room floor rather than in the swimming pool itself. So when you swim, wear a pair of water shoes or have them sitting by the side of the pool so that when you get out, you can easily put them on. Keep them on when you shower off and then stand on a towel when you change back into your clothes. Keeping your bare feet off the floor is your best protection.

Is there a special kind of lotion I should use because of my diabetes?

I have spent a lot of money trying to find a good moisturizing lotion for extremely dry skin, especially for my feet during the summer. I have not found anything that works as well as the stuff used on cow udders—Udder Butter, Bag Balm, or Corona Cream. We use it all the time in the hospital; the label is just covered so we do not offend patients. During the summer when I work outside all day, my feet get dry and calloused. After showering in the evening, I put Udder Butter on my feet and then put a pair of socks on (it will stain sheets). Nothing has worked better to prevent and treat cracks on my feet.

Am I sick because I'm high, or high because I'm sick?

Keeping your diabetes under control can be difficult even in the best of times. So it makes sense that when you are sick, diabetes management takes a little extra work. When you are sick, your body is under stress. The body responds to this stress by releasing the stress hormones—epinephrine, cortisone, and glucagon—to raise blood sugar levels. The idea is that releasing stored sugar into the bloodstream will convert more sugar into energy to help you heal. This works well if your body is able to produce insulin to help the sugar get to its destination. If your body cannot release extra insulin, then all it does is raise the blood sugar.

What you need to know is that you can plan on blood sugars rising during illness, even if you are not eating anything. Make a sick-day plan of action before you need it. Everyone on your diabetes team can help with this. Basically, you will go on treating your diabetes the same way you always have. However, there are a few rules that are good to know about sick days in relation to diabetes. Sick days might include flu or viruses, hospitalization for injury, illness, or surgery, or even having teeth pulled. A sick-day plan will help any time you are not functioning as usual and your body needs extra help.

Sick-Day Guidelines

Do not skip your diabetes medication if at all possible.
Remember that your blood sugars are going to be higher even if you
are not eating, so you still need help getting that sugar to its destination. Also know that high blood sugar levels interfere with the
body's immune system, which is helping you heal. You must keep
your blood sugars down to help you heal. This is why insulin may
be given temporarily when you are in the hospital. We know it
works. Pills may not be digested or absorbed as well, especially if
you are nauseated.

If you are taking diabetes pills, as soon as you can keep food
down, get your pills on board. It is okay if this takes several hours,
or even most of the day. What you don't want to do is stop taking
your medications. As soon as you can keep something in your
stomach, get back on schedule with your pills.

If you are on insulin, speak with your health care provider
about a sick-day insulin plan. Usually half of the long-lasting
insulin is given, and rapid-acting insulin is given every three or four
hours as needed for high blood sugars.

Check your blood sugars more often than usual. Blood
sugars can elevate quickly, especially if you become dehydrated.
Check at least four times a day if you use meal planning or pills to
control your diabetes, more often if you are on insulin. This way, if
you see your blood sugar climbing, you can let your physician know
before it is the middle of the night. People sometimes see glucose
levels of 200–300 when they are ill, but if levels are going above
300, let your physician know. Your health care professionals may
want to wait for a while, increase your medications, call in an
antibiotic, or even give you some insulin. Early intervention
prevents the need for hospitalization.

Check for urine ketones if you are taking insulin, you are
vomiting, and blood sugars are above 240 mg/dl. Ketones are the
waste product of fats being burned for energy instead of sugar,
which I will explain more fully with DKA. If you have moderate to
high ketones, call your doctor for help.

Drink plenty of fluids. Illness is a time when anyone can become dehydrated. Vomiting, diarrhea, and fever all decrease fluids needed for circulation and healing. When your blood sugars are running higher, you will also lose more urine. This makes you even more prone to dehydration. Try taking in at least half a cup of noncaloric fluid every hour when you are sick. This does not mean you have to get up every hour to drink, although that would help. Still, in a four-hour period, get in at least 2 cups of fluid. If you have a fever, double this amount. Fluids that work well for hydration without causing blood sugars to go up include water; hot or iced tea; broth; coffee; and sugar-free hot chocolate, soda, punch, or Jell-O.

Try to follow your meal plan. This is difficult to do when you feel fine, so why is it so important when you're sick? Well, your main goal is to prevent your cells from starving. The cells need sugar, which comes from food, to convert into energy to help you heal. Good nutrition is also needed for wound healing, keeping hydrated, fighting infection, and supplying your body with extra nutrients to rebuild strength. Even though all food groups are important, if we had to say "at least get this in," it would be carbo-hydrates, because they feed the cells first.

How can you take in enough carbohydrate if you cannot keep down anything solid? Simple. Use any fluid that has a high carbo-hydrate content. I could never understand as a child why I could have a regular Coke when I was sick, but when I was well I had to have the sugar-free Coke. The reason is that you are trying to replace the calories and carbohydrate from solid nutrition with the same amount of calories or carbohydrate in liquids, and the only way to do this is with high-carbohydrate liquids. If you are directed to have 45 grams of carbohydrate for a meal, but you can only keep liquids down, look at all the things you could have that would meet your needs:

1 can Coke or Sprite (39 g)	1 regular popsicle (30 g)
1 1/2 cups most juices (45 g)	1 cup (15 g) Gatorade
1 1/2 cups regular Jell-O (45 g)	3/4 cup sherbet (45 g)

A word of caution: Even though these liquids can fill your carbohydrate need, they have little nutrition or staying power. They are not recommended for regular use as a meal. If you need something in a semi-liquid form to replace a meal because of mouth surgery, diet restrictions, other illness, or simply a lack of appetite or time for a sit-down meal, there are better choices, such as

Carnation Instant Breakfast—regular, 1 pkg = 36 g
Carnation Instant Breakfast—sugar-free, 1 pkg = 22 g
Ensure, 1 can = 34 g
Glucerna, 1 can = 22 g
Boost, 1 can = 41 g
Chocolate milk—regular, 1 cup = 26 g
Chocolate milk—sugar-free, 1 cup = 18 g
Choice DM, 1 can = 28 g

Have a sick-day plan and a sick-day box. If you know that when you are sick the only thing that settles your stomach is Pepto-Bismol, Coke, or chicken soup, have some in a special place just for sick days. If you know that you throw up a lot when sick, have your physician prescribe something for nausea that you can keep on hand. Anything that you know works for you when you are sick is a good idea to have in a special place or box so that no one has to run out to get them.

Sick-Day Box Ideas

Regular Coke or Sprite   Clear broth
Saltine crackers   Thermometer
Tylenol or Aspirin   Cough syrup
Nausea medication   Cold or flu remedies
Diarrhea medication   Throat lozenges
Fast-acting insulin
Telephone numbers of your physician and nurse educator

See information on over-the-counter drugs below on p. 91.

Get plenty of rest. In this way, energy is used just for healing you.

Have accurate records of your blood sugar levels, ketones, fluid intake, and the medication you have taken. These records will save a lot of time in helping your physician figure out how to help you.

Have someone check on you frequently. This allows you to rest completely and let someone else be responsible for making sure you are okay.

Call Your Physician If:

- you are unable to keep down any fluids for 12–24 hours

- blood sugar levels are rapidly climbing or are not responding to insulin

- your urine shows moderate or high ketone levels

- you are having difficulty breathing, or chest or abdominal pain

- you are having trouble staying alert or are difficult to awaken

- you have a high fever

- your symptoms are worsening

- you have sudden weight loss

- any wound or extremity is red, hot, swollen, or draining

- if you are unsure about how to manage your diabetes

Over-the-Counter Medications

Most over-the-counter medications are fine to take with regard to diabetes, even though many of them may say something like "If you have diabetes or high blood pressure, check with your physician before use." There are two main reasons for this warning. First, using the product may have an effect on your blood sugar level; and second, it may aggravate existing complications of diabetes. If you are checking your blood sugar more frequently when you are ill, you may pick up on this. Many medications can affect the blood sugar, but not severely enough that you avoid taking them. However, the cautions on the label are very important if you have high blood pressure or other complications of diabetes. Certain medications may decrease the signs and symptoms of hypoglycemia, some may raise blood pressure, and some may disguise symptoms of complications. Decongestants may narrow blood vessels to help with congestion, but at the same time raise blood pressure or constrict vessels in other parts of the body. Weight-loss drugs should be taken cautiously. Many weight-loss drugs contain the herb ephedra, which acts like adrenaline. Ephedra may give you energy, but at the same time it raises your blood sugar, blood pressure, and heart rate. Read the labels; know why the cautions are there. If you are unsure about a certain medication, be sure to ask your physician or pharmacist for the safest and most accurate advice.

Hospitalization Help

Probably the best advice I can give you about being in the hospital is that nurses, and even physicians, will not understand the new way we do meal planning, the effects of medications or insulin, and most critically, the effect of high blood sugar on healing, especially wound healing. So let me give you some information to help during a hospitalization and some information to pass on to your health care providers.

First, you need to know that diabetes affects every single part of the body, every single cell in the body. So no matter what you are in the hospital for, diabetes is going to affect your recovery. People with diabetes have a higher risk for complications after surgery than anyone else, but it does not have to be that way. Aggressive blood sugar management is the best way to speed recovery and avoid additional complications. Tell your physician you want tight blood sugar control, even if that means taking insulin temporarily.

When blood sugar levels are above 200 mg/dl, the following conditions occur:

- Red blood cells lose their ability to deform. Deformability allows the red blood cells to adjust their shape to fit through the tiniest of capillaries, thus improving circulation.

- White blood cells lose their ability to find bacteria; the ability to kill the bacteria is impaired, and the bacteria are being fed by the high blood sugar.

- High blood sugars increase clotting time, which increases the risk for blood clots and vascular complications.

- Electrolyte imbalance and dehydration occur faster in patients with diabetes than in patients without diabetes.

- The rate of infection increases from 2% to 11%.

I do not know how many times I have argued with physicians who have told me that there is no need to worry about blood sugar levels until patients have recovered from surgery. The reasons above are only some of the effects of high blood sugar. The list could go on. The bottom line: If blood sugars are high, your recovery time takes longer, you are more at risk for complications from surgery, and wound healing and strength decrease. You need your blood sugar under control to recover from surgery.

When it comes to hospital personnel managing your diabetes, remember this: It has taken months to years for you to learn how to manage your diabetes. Most nurses will not have the education and knowledge you have about diabetes. Carbohydrate counting is especially new to nurses, because it is not usually taught in the nursing curriculum. Therefore, you may need to educate nurses about the meal plan you are on. For example, explain to them why you can have a regular Sprite when you are not eating anything solid. Be sure you get the medications in the right dose, the way you take them at home, if possible. Be patient with the nurses. Nurses, like doctors, have to keep track of hundreds of diseases and treatments. You are the expert on diabetes. Educate them.

For planned hospitalizations, I have a few recommendations that may help.

Have your glucose meter with you. In the hospital setting, different drugs and the effects of anesthesia can cause a variety of different symptoms and sensations, some of which mimic low blood sugar. If you have a meter with you, you can quickly check to see if you are low, whereas it sometimes takes the nurses quite a while to get to you. I also recommend having something with you to treat low blood sugars. As a floor nurse, I had times when I could not immediately respond to a call light because I was in the middle of another emergency or assignment. If you are having a low blood sugar, waiting for treatment can be scary. If you do treat for hypoglycemia, be sure to let your nurse know so that she can document it in your chart.

Have someone with you that knows how to manage diabetes. If you are having surgery or are ill enough that you cannot always help yourself, have someone stay with you that knows how to check your blood sugar and treat for hypoglycemia. Your support person can be sure you get needed snacks and medications, and can go out and get someone for help if necessary. The more your support person knows about your medications and diabetes treatment, the better.

Request that the diabetes nurse visit or make recommendations. If you are having planned surgery, make an appointment with your diabetes nurse educator before the surgery. Devise a medication and blood-monitoring plan, and arrange to see her while in the hospital if possible. If needed, have the diabetes educator talk with hospital personnel that will be taking part in your care.

Schedule surgeries to be first in the morning if possible and adjust medications accordingly. A lot of confusion and misunderstanding go along with surgery and what to do about your diabetes medications. The part often forgotten by patients and health care providers is that medication, especially insulin, is not just needed for food. You have all those counterregulatory hormones that are going to be released and a liver that is going to release extra sugar, since you are not eating. So even though you are in a fasting state, you will still need some medication. If you can schedule your surgery early in the morning, then you can take your oral medications as soon as you wake up from surgery and can tolerate fluids or semi-solids. If you have to wait until late in the afternoon for surgery, it is harder to know what to do with your medications because you will be going so long without eating. For some this would be a problem, for others not. If possible, put your surgery or procedure where it fits best in your schedule. If you take insulin, you will need a plan for how much and when to inject. Often we will still have you take your long-acting insulin (NPH, Lente, Ultralente, or glargine) as usual, or at least half of it. Blood sugars go high during surgery, and we need something on board to counteract the rise. Short-acting insulin won't be given before surgery except for what you need for a high blood sugar level. There are many ways to adjust insulin for surgery. The most important thing is to have some on board to prevent hyperglycemia.

Some medications, such as Glucophage, may need to be temporarily withheld while you receive certain diagnostic procedures, or if you are dehydrated, or your kidneys have been affected by your illness or surgery. This will eliminate the risk for toxicity of the drug.

Be sure all health care providers know you have diabetes. Someone may be performing surgery or a diagnostic procedure on you that you have never talked to before, especially anesthesiologists. Remind all health care providers that you have diabetes.

Have a list of your medications and doses. You are under a lot of stress when you enter the hospital, planned or unplanned. A list of your medications and the dosages will help eliminate the possibility of any medication being forgotten. If you are receiving meals and your medications have not been ordered, have your nurse call. You do not want to wait until your physician sees you next; that may be more than 24 hours.

You may have an IV with dextrose (sugar) in it. This procedure seems to go against everything we've said about keeping blood sugars down, but this is a common and safe practice. When we talked about meal planning for sick days, I showed you how to use regular soda pop in place of solid food for the purpose of getting some calories and carbohydrate in you. The IV with sugar does the same thing. If you cannot eat or drink, the only way to keep your cells fed and prevent starvation is to give you some sugar in your IV. As soon as you can tolerate liquids, the IV will be turned down or discontinued. Also, the amount of sugar or carbohydrate in most IV solutions is about 2.5–10 grams per 100 cc's of fluid. That is not much sugar when you consider you may only be getting 100 cc's an hour. If you feel your IV is causing trouble with your blood sugar, speak with your physician.

Know your rights. Usually you do not have to demand things aggressively in the hospital, but you will need to speak up for yourself. You know what it takes to manage your disease. And even though you are in a hospital setting, you are still in charge of your diabetes.

QUESTIONS

What is DKA or diabetic coma? Can adults develop this?

Diabetic ketoacidosis is a serious, life-threatening condition that typically occurs in patients with type 1 diabetes. It is the result of prolonged high blood sugars due to a lack of insulin, dehydration, and ketone production, which lead to an acid-base imbalance. Stomach pain and vomiting are classic symptoms of DKA. This vomiting leads to further dehydration and the inability of the body to circulate insulin and fluid to all the cells in the body. When the sugar gets to the cell doors and there is no insulin to let it in, the sugar level builds up in the bloodstream, and the cells that need sugar for fuel go hungry. Well, the cells know that if they cannot get sugar for fuel, they will have to find another source. The cells start to use another source of fuel from the body—fat. Fat does not require insulin to be pulled into the cell and burned for fuel. But this does cause a problem for the cell.

Imagine if you were instructed by a dietitian that all you could eat the rest of your life was shortening, lard, or butter. How well would you feel? Could you even get a spoonful of shortening swallowed without getting sick? Well, the cells feel the same way— eating all that fat makes the cell sick. And the way I explain it to my patients is that the cell throws up. What is the cell throwing up? Ketones.

Ketones are produced when fats have been burned for energy in place of sugar in the normal metabolic process. Why is this such a problem? When fats are burned at this unhealthy rate, they raise the body's acid level. A body cannot function with high levels of sugar and acid. This is what we call diabetic coma, or diabetic ketoacidosis. When the body is dehydrated, ketones are present, and the body is in an acidic state, the brain and other organs cannot function properly. Organs stop working, the brain shuts down, and the body falls into coma. This patient is in critical and immediate need of fluid for hydration, and then insulin. If we can catch ketone production early, we can prevent DKA or treat it at home with a sick-day plan of action.

HHS is a similar condition to DKA and is seen more often in adults with type 2 diabetes, although it is rare. HHS stands for extreme hyperglycemia (900–2000 mg/dl blood sugar), extreme dehydration, and thick dehydrated blood, but the patient is without ketones. The high blood sugars develop slowly and are tolerated longer. Excess blood sugars are excreted by the kidneys until dehydration is such that the kidneys can no longer function. The dehydration causes the blood to be more concentrated because there is not enough fluid to dilute or distribute the components. Some insulin is still being made in this condition, so the fat-burning process that we see in DKA is usually not present. Volume depletion leads to poor circulation and decreased cardiac output, which can be fatal.

Nothing can help this patient until there is rapid, precise, and timely rehydration. This condition is rare, seen more commonly in the elderly who live alone or in nursing homes. Their high blood sugar–caused decrease in level of consciousness may be attributed to their age, stroke, or other illnesses. Sometimes the elderly go untreated until they are found nonresponsive. This is why it is critical that you get plenty of fluid every day, but especially when you are ill.

I have to. I want to. I will!

(The emotional side of diabetes)

I read once that diabetes was one of the top causes of depression. A roommate at the time questioned how this could be true, when all you had to do was take your medication and eat right. After I got over the urge to throttle her, I tried to explain why diabetes can be so challenging. Diabetes is a 24-hour-a-day job, one you did not apply for. There are no vacations, no 15-minute breaks, no holidays, nor even time off for good behavior. It is a job that demands attention to details, timing, input and output, data collecting, and investigative thinking.

Everything you do—eating, exercising, working, sitting, sleeping, crying—changes your blood sugar. Even if you did the exact same thing every single day of your life, blood sugars levels might be different. Blood sugar levels are not always predictable. And there are no guarantees that if you do everything right, blood sugars will respond as we hoped they would. If you work very hard at bringing blood sugars into a near-normal range, you increase the risk of severe hypoglycemia. If you do not aim for tight control, you are at greater risk for the long-term complications of diabetes. Either direction sometimes feels like a trap.

Another hard part is that you did not apply for this job. You were delegated, assigned, given the opportunity, sentenced, or blessed with diabetes. No matter what attitude you have about it, it is still a challenge. Happily, it is a manageable challenge. And the more you work with it, the more you find tricks of the trade to help you cope and get on top. Taking steps to befriend your diabetes will ease some of the daily trials. Here are some of the ways I have chosen to deal with my own diabetes. Perhaps some of them will help you, as well.

Remember who you are. Diabetes does not change that. You are still the same person you were prior to being diagnosed with diabetes. You just have a chronic disease. Your reason for existence is not just to manage your diabetes, but to live life to the fullest, to love and to laugh. For the most part, you can continue to do what you like to do. Do not let diabetes stop you from being who you are.

Control the diabetes so it won't control you. When I was younger I used to always think to myself, "I have to eat on time, I have to exercise, I have to take my shots, and I have to check my blood," just because I had diabetes. At some point I was able to change my thinking to "I'm going to eat right, I'm going to exercise, and I'm going to check my blood and take my insulin, so that my diabetes won't control me." When we take a few daily steps to manage our diabetes, it will not have the power to prevent us from doing what we want to do in this life. A few minutes of self-care daily can add years to your life, whereas letting your diabetes manage itself will shorten your life considerably. Do not control it because you have to, *control it because you want to.*

Set small, achievable goals. If you take on every task of diabetes and try to change all your habits at once, it is over-whelming. Start by changing one thing, not everything. When you set smaller goals, they don't overwhelm you, and you are more likely to succeed. Instead of setting a goal to eat perfectly—and there is no such thing—set a goal not to have seconds or not to eat in the car. Make it something you can succeed in doing, then set another goal. One of the hardest goals people set is to lose weight. If your goal is to lose 50 pounds, even if you are successful, it will take a year or more to do it. For most people, it is hard to endure that long. If you set a goal to lose 5 pounds, you will succeed sooner, feel better about your ability to follow through with meal planning and exercise, and have more confidence in losing the next 5 pounds. Once you achieve several of your goals, congratulate or reward yourself in a positive way, then *set more goals.* It is easier to achieve your goals if you know what they are. So avoid setting vague or general goals, such as just "to take better care of yourself." Rather, set a goal for a specific behavior you can change to take better care of yourself. For example, "I will walk three times a week after lunch for 20 minutes."

Acknowledge that you do have choices. This gives you power. You can monitor your blood sugar or not, follow a meal plan or not, exercise or not exercise. Diabetes does not force you into doing these things. You always have a choice. Those who choose not to follow recommendations for good self-care later wish they did. So take control—make wise choices when it comes to your life with diabetes.

Take a stand on what you believe. Too many times I see patients with the attitude that "diabetes is a disease; therefore, I am sick." Because they believe this, they become sick. While it is true that diabetes is a disease, it does not make you sick unless you let it. You can still do everything you ever wanted. And you can feel good while you do it. Many people feel better than ever before because they are finally living a healthy lifestyle. Adopt the attitude that "diabetes will not change me," and then it will not.

Be realistic. Do not give diabetes more power than it ought to have. A close friend of mine has had diabetes for about nine years. She requires daily insulin injections and obviously should be checking blood sugars several times a day. Often she stops checking and stops taking her insulin. When I recently talked to her about her reasons for doing this, she said that it took too much time away from her family. As a result of this thinking, in one year she ended up in ICU six different times for a week or more. Today she struggles with all the complications of diabetes. Which is taking more time from her family? Several minutes a day to take her insulin and check a blood sugar, or more than six weeks in the hospital, plus a shorter, unhealthy life from avoiding the diabetes? Do not give your diabetes the power or permission to complicate your life. Take charge.

Find a good reason to have your diabetes. I still wish I did not have diabetes. And yet at the same time, my patients are always glad that I do because I can understand them more fully. I can speak from experience. I can say I understand, and they know that I do. I have also learned a lot about self-discipline and willpower—the constant need to keep working. If this book is helpful to only one person, then the experiences I have had with diabetes have been good for something. Maybe for you the diagnosis of diabetes was a turning point to a healthier life. Maybe diabetes puts you in touch with some of the good friends you have today. Maybe it just saves you time trying to decide which pop to get at McDonald's, because they only have one sugar-free drink. Crazy or not, find some good things about your diabetes.

Find tricks to make your diabetes regimen less time-consuming.

- **Get an extra meter.** Keep one in the bathroom so that while your blood sugar is counting down, you can brush your teeth, put in contact lenses, shave, dress, or shower. You do not have to sit and watch the meter; it will still give you a result when you get back to it.

- **Keep necessary equipment in a convenient, easy-to-access place** so that you can monitor or inject any time without feeling inconvenienced. I have a meter in almost every room of my house so that no matter where I am, I can check easily. I do not necessarily have my meters where everyone can see them, but when I see them I am reminded to check, and I do not mind it as much.

- **Put pills in a pill box** so that you don't have to open multiple containers morning and night, and so that you don't forget any.

- **Premix insulin syringes, if applicable.** R/NPH, 70/30 and 75/25 can be mixed and stored for short time periods, but not L, U, or R combinations. You can also purchase insulin pens that are convenient and easy to use.

- **Get all your prescriptions on the same refill schedule** so that you do not have to go to the pharmacy several different times a month. If your insurance has a mail-order pharmacy, use it! You can have three months worth of medication delivered all at once and at a better price.

- **Have a travel bag with all your diabetes supplies,** except insulin and maybe your pills, already packed, so that you can grab it at the last minute and know you will have what you need. Include snack items, low blood sugar treatments, an extra meter with test strips, lancets, syringes, and ketone strips.

- **Use a meter with a memory.** Just do not forget to download it or look at your numbers frequently. Looking at your glucose numbers only when you see a physician is not often enough.

Keep a sense of humor. This has helped me tremendously. Even if you scream and then laugh about screaming, it somehow helps. There is nothing funny about diabetes itself, or any disease. But usually there are parts of the management that can be looked at with a smile to ease the difficulty of it.

In sum, diabetes is manageable. Find some creative ways to help you manage it so that it does not interfere as much. Talk to as many people as you can who also have diabetes. They can tell you what works for them.

QUESTIONS

How can I help my friends understand diabetes?

Even if you have had diabetes for 20 years, it can still be difficult to understand. So trying to teach others about it can be frustrating, even when they are totally interested. They do not have the exposure to it that you do. For most people, diabetes means you cannot eat sugar. It takes years for new information to make it to the ears of the public, and years to change old ways of thinking. When the opportunity is right, educate those whom you would like to be a support to you. Be prepared for people to respond differently than you expect them to.

When some people know you are dealing with a loss or an illness, they share what they know about that illness, and diabetes does not always bring the most pleasant memories. People mean well, but what they say does not always come across that way. They will share their memories of a grandparent, aunt, uncle, or a friend of a friend who had serious complications of diabetes. You will also hear from people about miracle cures, herbs, or vitamins that will replace the need for insulin. Unfortunately, there is no replacement for insulin, period.

Do not let these people challenge what you know. Be a wise consumer. Their ideas can be mighty convincing, but to be safe, check their advice out with your diabetes educator. You will also have people who act like policemen, nicknamed "diabetes police." They tell you what you should or should not do, what you should and should not eat, and it seems like they are always watching your every move. They mean well, they just have not been educated enough to know how to really help. Finally, know that there will be friends who will try to understand, and there will be those who *don't want to understand.* Diabetes may scare them or remind them of someone. For some, it is no concern of theirs.

Diabetes is nothing to be ashamed of, but you do not have to tell everyone. Choose to tell those who can support your efforts and have a concern for your well-being. In the work, school, or driving setting, you do have a responsibility to be safe. This means choosing someone to know about your diabetes, having an emergency plan, and knowing when you should not be driving or using equipment that could be dangerous. The world is an easier place when people you care about know you have diabetes. Their knowing about your diabetes also gives them the opportunity to be a support to you.

If I don't feel sick, how can high blood sugars hurt me?

(Long-term complications of diabetes)

Why do complications occur, and what are they? With improvements in medical care, we are living longer and this may be one of the reasons we still see complications of diabetes. The longer we live with diabetes, the more we are at risk for complications from it. As a child, I never understood threats such as "If you eat that, you'll go blind" or "You'll have to get your legs cut off if you don't take your shot." These threats did not mean anything because in my mind, I was not hurting and I felt fine, so how could something bad be happening? I had skipped my shots and gone off my diet multiple times before, and I could still walk and still see, so the threats did not carry any validity.

Furthermore, I did not know what my diabetes had to do with losing a leg or my vision. To me, diabetes was about avoiding sugar. I did not understand that my control as I grew up would affect my risk for complications as an adult. I did not know there was something I could do about it. And bottom line, I did not understand. I was told about all the problems my diabetes could cause, but nobody explained why.

Had someone explained these things to me, I might have tried harder to do what I had been told to do. Complications from diabetes come on over time, and damage has often started before we realize something is wrong. The belief that "as long as I feel well I must be well" does not hold true for the complications of diabetes; they come on quietly. Let me explain in the simplest way I know to help you understand how complications occur. This is not a medical book explanation, but it is a simple analogy of what is going on in the body when blood sugars are allowed to run even mildly high.

Blood Sugars and Complications

Picture the freeways leading to Salt Lake City. They have the job of carrying thousands of people in thousands of cars to specific destinations. Compare the freeways to the blood vessels in the body, in that the vessels have the job of carrying multiple forms of nutrition to specific destinations. The cars on the freeway can be compared to the pieces of nutrition that are in the blood. Both have a destination—the cars need to get to Salt Lake City, and the nutrition needs to get to every cell in the body. To get them to their destination, both also have a path, the freeway or vascular system of the body. Let us say that our destination is a Jazz basketball game at the Delta Center.

First you need to understand what makes up the blood. Too often we see it as that darn red drop of fluid that we can never squeeze enough of from our finger. With all due respect, however, blood is one of the most precious, nutritious fluids we have on the earth. Blood contains the nutrients we need to maintain life. It is made up of red blood cells, which carry oxygen and facilitate the passage of nutrition through small narrow vessels throughout the body. White blood cells fight off bacteria and infection and dispose of it. Sugar in the blood feeds the cells, and insulin in the blood helps the sugar get into the cells. Platelets help our blood clot so that we do not bleed too much. Electrolytes keep our heart and muscles contracting and relaxing as they should, and different forms of fat keep us flexible and serve as extra energy. The list could go on. The blood is packed with nutrition, just as the freeway is packed with cars during rush-hour traffic.

When blood sugar levels run higher than normal, the red blood cells become sticky and stiff. This is because sugar in excess permanently attaches to parts of the red blood cell—sugar coating them. What would something sticky in the bloodstream do? Logically, it would gum things up and slow circulation down. I like to compare sticky red blood cells to a cop car on the freeway or an oversized semi-truck or even a slow car in the fast lane. These vehicles force us to slow down! If we assess both scenarios, can we get to Salt Lake City even if there are slow cars, cops, and oversized semi-trucks? Yes. It may take a little longer, and we may be annoyed, but we can still get there. The same holds true for the nutrition units in the presence of sticky red blood cells. For the most part they can still get to their destination, but interference has begun. It does not stop there, unfortunately.

When sugar attaches to the red blood cell for an extended period, it hardens and crystalizes. Remember that red blood cells are supposed to be flexible and slippery so that they can slide through the tiniest of vessels. Now they are hard, and as they flow through the vessels they scratch or damage the lining of the vessels, kind of like a large truck dragging machinery as it goes down the road, making potholes in it. Potholes in the road damage the cars that hit them. In the vessels, the damaged parts trap nutrition and waste products as these flow by. Your body knows that nutrition stuck in the potholes will never reach its destination, so the body fills the pothole with cholesterol.

Cholesterol paves over the damaged area, just as gravel is used to fill the potholes in the road narrowing vessels and decreasing circulation. We hear often that high fat levels cause hardening of the arteries, and this is true, but high blood sugars contribute to it as well. You can also liken these damaged areas in the vessels to construction areas on the freeway. Once again, the cars can still make it to Salt Lake City, but now there are construction and road closures on top of slow cars, trucks, and police cars. People are starting to have second thoughts about going to Salt Lake City; for some it is not worth the hassle. The same thing is starting to happen with the circulatory process. Nutrition is losing some of its "drive" to get to its destination. The problem goes further.

If all the red blood cells in the body are sticky, that means that everything they touch will become sticky as well. This stickiness forms on every vessel in the body, narrowing the passageway. I liken this to going from a three-lane road to a two-lane road with construction, potholes, cops, slow cars, and semi-trucks. More and more people are deciding not to fight the traffic or the interference. Nutrition is also having a difficult time getting to its destination, and much of it is not getting there at all.

When blood sugar levels consistently run high, so do cholesterol and triglyceride levels. High fat levels also narrow the vessels. Now we are looking at going to Salt Lake City on a one-lane road, with construction, potholes, cops, slow cars, and semi-tucks. Who wants to go now? Very few will even try. Picture the same thing happening in your body. Where the vessels are big, circulation still gets through. But where the vessels are small, the road begins to close. Circulation decreases or is halted, and that part of the body becomes malnourished and damaged.

So where are the smallest vessels in the body? In the feet and fingers, eyes, kidneys, and heart. These are where the most common complications of diabetes occur, but every part of the body is affected. These complications rarely develop suddenly. Instead, they complicate your life by creating pain and disability. I hear a lot of people say they are going to do whatever they want, eat whatever they want, and let the diabetes take them when it is time.

The problem with this plan is that poorly managed diabetes does not "take you" all at once, it takes you a toe at a time. So every little effort you make to improve your diabetes management will help prevent or delay complications in the years ahead. Let's look at the specific parts of the body that are damaged most frequently by poorly controlled diabetes.

Cardiovascular System

The heart actually has the largest blood vessels in the body, so why is it damaged? First of all, it is the job of the heart to pump the thick, sticky blood through all the narrowed vessels in the body. That is like canoeing in Jell-O compared with canoeing in water. The heart also has many small vessels that feed and nourish it. When blood sugars are high, they do not get the circulation they need. So not only are we asking the heart to work twice as hard, we are depriving it of nutrition to give it strength. **Cardiovascular Disease** is the most common cause of death in people with diabetes. But there are prevention and treatment strategies that have been proven effective. We tend to be more sensitive to lower levels of blood fats and cholesterol; this is why we are given specific recommendations for these blood fat levels. People with diabetes do not always have the normal symptoms associated with a heart attack or heart damage. Hence it is critical to have regular checkups that assess heart activity.

Vision Problems

Retinopathy, macular edema, glaucoma, and cataracts are the more common eye disorders related to diabetes. Circulation to the eye works a bit like watering the lawn with a garden hose. Water is carried by various hoses to different parts of your yard, just as various vessels in the retina carry blood to the different parts of your eye. If there is a kink in the hose, there is no circulation past the kink, and behind the kink, pressure builds up. If there is a weak spot in the hose, it bursts and leaks water.

The same thing happens in your eye when you have retinopathy. The blood, unable to circulate to the small vessels in the eye, builds up, causing excessive pressure. High blood sugars may have also weakened the vessels, so when the pressure builds up, the vessel bursts, causing blood to spill into the back of the eye. Once again, your body knows that where there are damaged vessels in the eye, there will be no circulation. Attempting to restore circulation, the eye grows new vessels but these new vessels are very fragile and break easily, so the leaking gets worse, eventually leading to vision loss. Retinopathy is not life-threatening, but it is sight-threatening. And vision loss is a threat to the quality of our life.

The macula is the part of the eye responsible for detailed vision. When fluid or blood leaks out of weak vessels in this particular area, there is swelling or macular edema, which interferes with the ability to adjust or focus on things. Glaucoma also occurs more frequently with diabetes. Fluid in the back of your eye helps your eyes keep their shape. In glaucoma, the fluid behind the eye builds up and has no place to go. This increased pressure decreases the circulation to the optic nerve and causes damage. This nerve damage may result in the muscles not being able to function properly, paralysis, or inability to coordinate eye movement. Cataracts also occur more often, causing a cloudiness on the lens of the eye, which obscures vision.

Eye disease is typically progressive, and there are usually no symptoms until damage has occurred. You may have 20/20 vision yet one day have complete vision loss due to a hemorrhage. This is the reason a yearly eye exam is so important. An eye doctor will be able to see the changes occurring before vision is at risk. Laser surgery can destroy the abnormal vessels in the eye and prevent their regrowth.

Foot and Leg Complications

Amputations and ulcers, especially in the feet, are more frequent in patients with poorly controlled diabetes. Decreased circulation to feet and legs leads to damage and loss of nerve function. The nerves lose their ability to sense pain, pressure, touch, or temperature correctly, which results in tingling and numbness of the feet and toes (fingers, too). This condition is called *peripheral neuropathy*. The decrease in sensation may lead to abnormal weight bearing and walking. The muscles may not be able to support the bony structures of the foot, and pressure sores develop over bones. You are more likely to injure your feet. So you have poor circulation, nerve damage, and an inability to tell when you have been injured. You have the conditions for ulcers that are very difficult to heal. These injuries go untreated when you do not know you have them. High blood sugars feed bacteria and interfere with the white blood cell's ability to destroy bacteria. So anytime there is a break in the skin, infection can result and be difficult to manage or to treat.

If you already have numbness in your feet, is there any point to controlling blood sugars? Absolutely. Numbness and burning in the feet are signs that nerves have been damaged. Evidence has shown that nerves, when only damaged, can learn to transmit messages through different pathways. If your feet are so completely numb that you cannot tell where they are because you cannot feel them, managing your blood sugars most likely will not get any sensation back. But it can prevent the numbness and nerve damage from spreading farther up your leg. And controlling your blood sugars will give your damaged nerves and your immune system a fighting chance to help your feet stay healthy.

Kidney Disease

The kidneys have the job of being filters for the blood. They decide what should stay circulating and what should be taken out as waste products or urine. When the kidneys have spent too much time filtering excess sugar from the blood, they become tired and damaged. They can no longer tell what is good and what is bad, or what should stay and what should go. Because of this, some waste products will remain in the blood, and some nutrition, such as protein, is let out into the urine. This is what we call kidney disease or *nephropathy*. Research has shown that early detection and treatment can prevent or delay the onset and progression of kidney disease. ACE inhibitor medications have been found both to lower blood pressure and give extra protection to the kidneys.

Nerve Damage and Disease

Autonomic neuropathy occurs when there is nerve damage affecting the automatic processes in your body such as heart rate or sweating, so they do not work as they should. The stomach may not process food correctly. The heart rate or blood pressure does not speed up or slow down in response to exercise, exertion, rest, standing, or sitting. Autonomic neuropathy also contributes to the absence of chest pain with a heart attack, and can cause sweating at inappropriate times or in specific areas, leaky bladder, pupils that do not constrict or dilate as needed, sexual dysfunction, and decreased ability to sense an infection or hypoglycemia.

So What's the Good News?

Believe it or not, there is some good news. The whole process of long-term complications started with sticky red blood cells. The good news is that red blood cells only live two to three months. That means that in three months of keeping your blood sugar levels nearer to normal, you have a whole new set of unsticky red blood cells. This turnover eliminates the cops, slow cars, and semi-trucks from the freeway, and prevents further damage to the road. When blood sugar levels come down, the stickiness decreases on the walls of the arteries and veins, and triglyceride and cholesterol levels are reduced. So where lanes of traffic were closed, we now have open roads. Where damage has been done, we may not be able to repair it, but with improved control, we can prevent further complications and slow or stop the progress of any existing ones. Keeping blood sugars close to normal is the best way to prevent complications. Unlike genetics, age, or sex, it is the one component we have some control over.

QUESTIONS

Should I worry about taking good care of my diabetes when I am elderly and already have some complications?

Absolutely! Even if you do not live long enough to develop long-term complications of diabetes, the short-term complications of hyperglycemia can make you miserable. High blood sugars lead to decreased energy, frequent yeast infections, incontinence, poor wound healing, insomnia, bad moods, and scads of other medical problems. If setting goals that apply to years down the road doesn't work for you, perhaps your goals should be to live symptom-free and feeling good for the time you do have. Nobody knows how long that will be. We do not want to just prevent complications. We want to improve your quality of life today!

Chapter 14

Does this disease come with a guarantee?

Taking good care of your diabetes does not guarantee that you will not have complications. On the other hand, we do know that if you do not take control of it, you are guaranteed to have complications. Play your best hand. Even if complications from diabetes do come, they will be more easily controlled and will come much later in life.

I have heard it said that diabetes is 99% patient-managed and 1% physician-managed. I believe this. You are in charge of your diabetes 24 hours a day, 365 days a year. But that does not mean you have to do it alone. Use your physician as a guidance counselor. Empower him or her to help you. Keep a record book of your glucose numbers and insist that your health care providers look at them. If they do not know how to interpret blood sugars or do not think it is necessary, find a physician who does.

Create a diabetes team with your physician, nurse educator, counselor, dietitian, and exercise physiologist. Include your friends and family members on your team as well. Working with your diabetes team can help you stay motivated and help you get back on the right track if you have lost motivation. When you need help, you will feel more comfortable calling a nurse or physician if you know them well and they know you.

Recommended Tests

The American Diabetes Association offers guidelines for tests other than glucose levels that should be done in order to prevent or delay the complications of diabetes. Review these with your physician. The guidelines are there for a reason—to help you prevent avoidable complications. Recommendations from the ADA start with A, B, C:

A1C. An A1C test is a measurement of your overall glucose control for the previous two- to three-month period. It is an average and takes into account the good days and the bad. To help prevent complications, have an A1C done two to four times yearly and aim for 7.0 or less.

Blood pressure. High blood pressure, even mild elevations, puts you at increased risk for heart disease, retinopathy, and kidney disease. It is the leading cause of stroke and heart attack. The recommendation for blood pressure for adults with diabetes is less than (<)130/80.

Cholesterol. There is good (HDL) and bad (LDL) cholesterol in our body. If you go to a health fair to have your cholesterol level measured, and the result is one number, this is total cholesterol or a measurement of all the good and bad fats combined. For adults with diabetes total cholesterol should be less than (<)180.

LDL (lethal, or lousy, fats). These bad fats contribute to cholesterol buildup on the walls of arteries, which increases the risk of coronary artery disease. So you want your LDL level to be as **low** as possible. You want a low level of lethal, lousy fats. The ideal recommendation for adults is an LDL lower than 100, especially in women. Studies have shown that women who have a high LDL level are at the greatest risk for coronary artery disease or damage to the arteries that feed and nourish the heart.

HDL (healthy or happy fats). HDLs are good fats that are low in cholesterol and decrease the risk of coronary artery disease. So the more you have of them, the better. You should have a **high** amount of healthy, happy fats. The recommendation is greater than (>)35 for men and greater than (>)45 for women.

Triglycerides. These are additional forms of stored fats that can be broken down for energy. High levels of triglycerides contribute to a painful, destructive disease of the pancreas called *pancreatitis.* Adult levels should be less than (<)200.

Weight management. If you are overweight, even modest weight loss (10–15 pounds) will help improve blood sugar levels, lower blood pressure, and improve cholesterol levels. Work toward your desired weight as set by you, your dietitian, and your physician.

Foot exam. The best way to treat a foot problem is to prevent it. Take your shoes and socks off when you see your physician, so that he or she cannot help but see your feet. Do this at least twice yearly during routine checkups and as needed. Set a goal to have no foot ulcers or infections and to take preventive measure for foot deformities.

Dilated eye exam. This is not a test to see whether you need glasses. In a dilated eye exam, an ophthalmologist puts drops into your eyes that make the pupils dilate. With the pupils dilated, the eye doctor can look with a bright light and see the blood vessels in the back of your eye. If there are swollen or leaky vessels, they can be treated before they cause vision loss. If you wait until vision is lost, there may be little that can be done to restore even partial vision. Just as in kidney disease, there are no symptoms until it is too late. But with a yearly eye exam, problems can be found early and treated. Here is a complication you have a lot of control over. It is recommended that you have a dilated eye exam when you are diagnosed with diabetes, yearly thereafter in adults, and yearly in children starting five years after diagnosis. If you do need to be assessed for glasses, it is a good idea to wait until your blood sugars have stabilized for at least a month or so, because your vision will change. At that time, you may find that you have bought glasses that you do not need.

Microalbumin. Microalbumin is the smallest particle of protein we can measure in the urine. Protein present in the urine indicates that the kidneys have been damaged by diabetes. As filters, they may be losing their ability to decide what should stay in the body and what should be gotten rid of. You should not have protein in your urine. Be aware that there are no symptoms of diabetic kidney disease. Nothing will alert you to damage occurring until the damage is irreversible. Since microalbumin is the smallest amount of protein we can measure, if we catch it early, there is a lot we can do to prevent the progression of kidney disease. This should be tested yearly, and the desired goal is negative or less than (<)30.

Flu shot. Because of the severity of the flu, it is recommended that everyone with diabetes, adults and children, receive a flu shot prior to the cold and flu season. It is not that you are at greater risk for the flu, but if you do get it, your diabetes will aggravate the healing process.

These tests or exams are recommended to keep you healthy. They are critical in detecting and preventing complications. Abnormal results will show up in these tests before you have any symptoms. If you catch abnormalities early, they can be treated more easily and the progression of the complication can be slowed or even stopped. Do not just ask or encourage your physician to run these tests, insist on it!

Chapter 15

What to do when you're tired of doing all you're doing.

People often ask what the hardest part about being diabetic is for me. It probably depends on the day, but I think one of the hardest parts has been working toward certain goals. This is because even when I make them, I cannot stop doing the things that got me there. The work is not over. I can succeed at getting my A1C in a desired range, but then my work is not done. I still have to eat right, check my blood sugars, and exercise. When do I get a break, without it affecting my A1C? The truth is: never. Sometimes that is a hard bite to chew. I think having diabetes for 27 years makes this reality even more frustrating. Diabetes is not fair, not easy, not convenient, not cheap—and it is not going to go away. So now what? What do you do when you have had it, you are overwhelmed, and you just need a break? I don't have all the answers, but here is a plan.

Understand that you are trying to manage a disease that isn't predictable. Sometimes I think diabetes should be called Murphy's Disease, because so many of Murphy's Laws apply to it. Murphy's Laws for diabetes would include (1) just when you think you have it figured out, it changes again; (2) diabetes creates its own rules, but sticks to no rules; (3) diabetes is different in everyone; (4) every doctor will treat diabetes differently, so whom do you listen to? and (5) with diabetes, there is never any "always." The most predictable thing about diabetes is that it is unpredictable. Give yourself credit for everything you do to manage it.

Step back and look at the whole picture. One high blood sugar or an extra meal is not worth your throwing in the towel. Cut yourself some slack and allow yourself to be human. Deal with setbacks and move on. Start again tomorrow, start with the next meal, start right now, and reevaluate your goals. Reaffirm to yourself that your diabetes should not prevent you from doing everything you ever wanted to do. Often the biggest difference after diabetes is the lack of spontaneity. If you decide at the last minute to take off and go skiing, you do not need to pack just your ski gear, but your diabetes gear as well. I joke with the parents of young children that they have gotten rid of the diaper bag, but now they have a diabetes bag. The positive thing here is that by planning ahead or taking that diabetes bag with you, you are prepared for any problem that might arise, and you can treat it without it interfering with your plans.

Evaluate your expectations. Are they realistic? Are your expectations possible? Are you pushing yourself so hard that you are becoming angry or resentful of your diabetes? Again, set goals that you can accomplish, acknowledge your successes, and then work up to more challenging goals. Do not expect perfection in any aspect of your life. When you make a mistake or have a "bad diabetes day," allow yourself to learn from the experience. Instead of telling yourself off, decide what you will do differently next time.

Assess your barriers. What are you telling yourself about diabetes or your ability to manage it? Have you told yourself that it takes too much time or costs too much? Do your cultural beliefs contradict diabetes recommendations, or do you fear others finding out that you have diabetes? Do you feel like it is too late to change old habits? Are you afraid to succeed? Explore any beliefs that prevent you from taking the best care of yourself, then compromise if necessary. Any change you make, no matter how small, can only help your diabetes health.

Avoid "can't" comments. You can—you just have not yet.

Avoid "always" or "never" statements. Sometimes you do monitor blood sugar regularly or do follow your meal plan. Do not discount what you have done and can do.

Have a sense of humor. There is nothing funny about having a disease, but it helps to laugh about its management, because laughter eases the stress of it. In one of my classes, I mentioned how you could have a regular Coke when you were sick and could not keep anything solid down. Suddenly several hands went up in the back of the room. The young men explained that they were feeling sick all of a sudden and needed to go get a Coke. The people in class all had a good laugh, and it helped lighten the mood.

Focus on what you have done right. Everyone makes mistakes; what can you learn from the ones you have made? If your blood sugar is high, treat it and then focus on the fact that you took care of it, not that you had it. High blood sugars happen. Once you treat them, they are no longer an issue. If you frequently forget to take your medications, make a plan so that it is easier to remember. When you find solutions to problems like this, you are not so hard on yourself.

Stay educated. The more you know about diabetes, the more empowered you are to make educated decisions in its management. Attend a diabetes class. Knowledge does not make you take better care of yourself, but it gives you the power to if that is what you want. Without education, motivation has no place to go.

Don't let other people's attitude of "this is great and easy" fool you. Their management is not perfect, although their denial skills may be good. Do not set yourself up to fail by telling yourself you should be as good as someone else. We all have our difficult days. I used to believe that as long as I was not having low blood sugars, my control was great and easy. The reason, however, that I never ran too low was because, for many years, I ran too high. I was not high enough to feel lousy, but high enough not to have lows. The absence of extreme highs or lows is not necessarily an indicator of good control. I have also found that people who think their diabetes is in great control do not know what that really means. Do we ever really control our diabetes? Or is it more accurate to say we can manage it?

Visit your MD frequently. This lets the doctor know of your dedication to taking steps to improve your management. Again, if problems do arise, they will be detected sooner and will be more easily treated. It is much easier to prevent a complication than to treat one.

Cut yourself some slack. There is no such thing as a perfect patient, perfect person with diabetes, or perfect person, for that matter. Allow yourself to have good days and rough days, days you feel in control and days when your diabetes takes control. Maybe it would help to look at your diabetes as if it were a child. As adults we try to teach children right from wrong and how to behave; we try to control them. But children also have minds of their own, and sometimes they just have to do what *they* want, not what *you* want. Just like the child, sometimes our diabetes seems to do what it wants. And maybe you just need to do what you want rather than what the diabetes wants you to do. When you have done what you need to do to and you're ready to start again, review the skills you have to bring the situation back in order.

Set up a support network. Surround yourself with people who care about you and your diabetes. Sometimes you can hang on to them when you have a hard time hanging on for yourself.

Help someone else with diabetes. Often you will find that in helping others, you will find ways to help yourself as well. When I talk with people that have diabetes, the ideas and experiences we share give me more energy and desire to take better care of myself. And not only that, I am reminded that I am not alone. Seventeen million people have diabetes, and they all have some of the same fears, concerns, and hopes that I do.

Subscribe to a reputable diabetes magazine. *Diabetes Forecast* features articles on the tricks of the trade, how to get up when you are down, and how to stay motivated. It has pages of carbohydrate counting ideas, meal planning help, and exercise help. And the articles are written on your level, not a physician's level. The authors write about real life!

Job share. Find a friend, spouse, roommate, or coworker that can occasionally help with a certain task of your diabetes so that you can have a temporary break from that task. I had a young patient who just could not, would not, check his blood sugar before dinner. He did not mind all the other checks he had to do, but for some reason the dinnertime blood check just did not work for him. Together, we worked out a plan for his sister to monitor his dinnertime blood sugar. He did not have to get up and go anywhere. She would come to him, and all he had to do was hold out a finger. This approach decreased his anger toward his diabetes, allowed his sister to do something for him, and still accomplished the goal of getting a blood sugar level. You do not have to do it all alone. Inform support people of your needs and how they can help you.

Develop a hobby. Diabetes can be time-consuming, so be sure and find things to do that you enjoy in the time away from diabetes.

See a therapist for chronic illness counseling. Even though we cannot talk our diabetes away, sometimes talking about it does make it easier. Getting help with your diabetes does not mean you cannot cope or do it on your own, it means you are taking steps to help you manage it the best you can.

Give yourself credit for living a long time with a chronic disease and the accomplishments you have been able to make with it. Take a day at a time or even a meal at a time. You did not ask for the extra workload of diabetes, but you are doing it. Good for you!

Acknowledge even the smallest of achievements. Be proud of those holes in your fingers (or forearms or earlobes or thigh)! You are taking care of you, and that is the most important thing.

Positive self talk. Talk up to yourself, not down. "I'm high, and I treated it," rather than "I'm high, I failed."

Acknowledge your feelings. Diabetes definitely is not easy. There will be good days and bad days—and good days. What made the good days good and the bad days rough? We do not always know. Sometimes I ask my coworkers not to mention one thing about diabetes to me. Well, when you work in a diabetes clinic, that can be pretty hard to do. It is also hard to troubleshoot or problem solve on the rough days. Wait for a good day, then look back and use that information to make different plans.

What do you want to do with your diabetes? This is a tough question. Life deals us challenges every day. In a sense, you were "blessed" with diabetes. What are you going to do with it? I had to face a lot of challenges growing up; diabetes was only one of them. I made a declaration of self from a song I heard that helped me cope with my diabetes.

If there's a mountain I need to climb,
Give me that mountain, I'll make it mine.

Diabetes was one of my mountains. Somehow, find a way to make its management worth it for you.

And finally, what can diabetes do *for you?* Another tough question. It takes a lot of work and time to manage diabetes. So what can it do for you? It gave me a career opportunity—an opportunity to share from my own experiences. Not everyone will have these same opportunities, but there are others. Diabetes that is well cared for can make you one of the healthiest people on earth. You have learned about how the body works and what it needs to function best, and you are doing something about it.

Too many people believe that disease only happens to others. They do not take the opportunity to develop healthy lifestyles. They may not have diabetes, but they sure are unhealthy. The exercise physiologist I work with tells our patients that the healthiest way to live life is to get a chronic disease and to take good care of it.

I am healthy today, and I make healthy choices because of my diabetes—and look what it is doing for me. You can do it too!

Index

About the American Diabetes Association

The American Diabetes Association is the nation's leading voluntary health organization supporting diabetes research, information, and advocacy. Its mission is to prevent and cure diabetes and to improve the lives of all people affected by diabetes. The American Diabetes Association is the leading publisher of comprehensive diabetes information. Its huge library of practical and authoritative books for people with diabetes covers every aspect of self-care— cooking and nutrition, fitness, weight control, medications, complications, emotional issues, and general self-care.

To order American Diabetes Association books: Call 1-800-232-6733.
Or log on to http://store.diabetes.org

To join the American Diabetes Association: Call 1-800-806-7801.
www.diabetes.org/membership

For more information about diabetes or ADA programs and services:
Call 1-800-342-2383. E-mail: AskADA@diabetes.org or log on to www.diabetes.org

To locate an ADA/NCQA Recognized Provider of quality diabetes care in your area:
www.ncqa.org/dprp/

To find an ADA Recognized Education Program in your area: Call 1-888-232-0822.
www.diabetes.org/recognition/education.asp

To join the fight to increase funding for diabetes research, end discrimination, and improve insurance coverage: Call 1-800-342-2383. www.diabetes.org/advocacy

To find out how you can get involved with the programs in your community:
Call 1-800-342-2383. See below for program Web addresses.

- *American Diabetes Month:* Educational activities aimed at those diagnosed with diabetes—month of November. www.diabetes.org/ADM
- *American Diabetes Alert:* Annual public awareness campaign to find the undiagnosed— held the fourth Tuesday in March. www.diabetes.org/alert
- *The Diabetes Assistance & Resources Program (DAR):* Diabetes awareness program targeted to the Latino community. www.diabetes.org/DAR
- *African American Program:* Diabetes awareness program targeted to the African American community. www.diabetes.org/africanamerican
- *Awakening the Spirit: Pathways to Diabetes Prevention & Control:* Diabetes awareness program targeted to the Native American community. www.diabetes.org/awakening

To find out about an important research project regarding type 2 diabetes:
www.diabetes.org/ada/research.asp

To obtain information on making a planned gift or charitable bequest:
Call 1-888-700-7029. www.diabetes.org/ada/plan.asp

To make a donation or memorial contribution: Call 1-800-342-2383.
www.diabetes.org/ada/cont.asp